Visit our website

to find out about other books from Churchill Livingstor
and our sister companies in Harcourt Health Sciences

Register free at

www.harcourt-international.com

and y

- the
  pro

- the
  new

- new

- info
  com
  Mo

You w
inform

Visit t

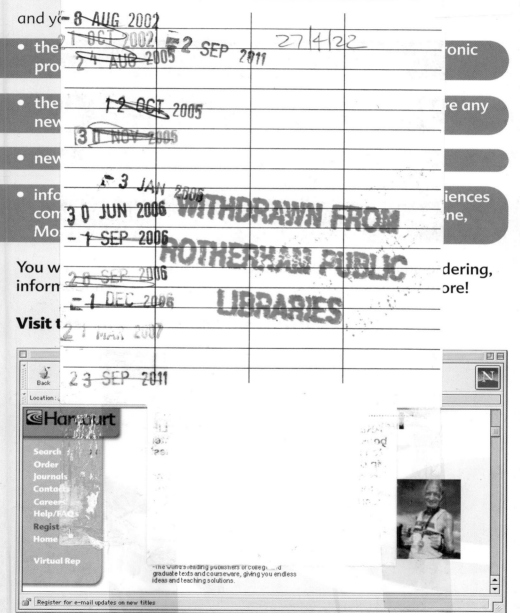

Back

Location :

Harcourt

Search
Order
Journals
Contacts
Careers
Help/FAQs
Register
Home

Virtual Rep

-the world's leading publishers of college and
graduate texts and courseware, giving you endless
ideas and teaching solutions.

Register for e-mail updates on new titles

Harcourt
Health Sciences

Data Questions for the
MRCPCH
Part 2

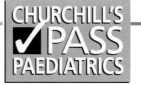

Commissioning Editor: Ellen Green
Project Development Manager: Barbara Simmons
Project Controller: Nancy Arnott
Designer: Judith Wright

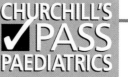

Data Questions
for the
MRCPCH
Part 2

J.L. Robertson

MB ChB MRCPCH
Staff Paediatrician
Wirral Hospital NHS Trust
Wirral, Merseyside, UK

A.P. Hughes

MB ChB MRCPCH
Consultant Paediatrician
Wirral Hospital NHS Trust
Wirral, Merseyside, UK

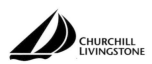

EDINBURGH LONDON NEW YORK PHILADELPHIA ST LOUIS SYDNEY TORONTO 2001

CHURCHILL LIVINGSTONE
An imprint of Harcourt Publishers Limited

© Harcourt Publishers Limited 2001

◑ is a registered trademark of Harcourt Publishers Limited

First published 2001

ISBN 0443 064741

British Library Cataloguing in Publication Data
A catalogue record for this book is available from the British Library

Library of Congress Cataloging in Publication Data
A catalog record for this book is available from the Library of
Congress

Medical knowledge is constantly changing. As new information
becomes available, changes in treatment, procedures, equipment and
the use of drugs become necessary. The editors/authors/contributors
and the publishers have, as far as it is possible, taken care to ensure
that the information given in this text is accurate and up to date.
However, readers are strongly advised to confirm that the
information, especially with regard to drug usage, complies with the
latest legislation and standards of practice.

The
publisher's
policy is to use
**paper manufactured
from sustainable forests**

Typeset by IMH(Cartrif), Loanhead, Scotland
Printed in Spain

Preface

This book has come about as a result of a simple request from one of our SHOs. In preparing for the written section of the MRCPCH Part 2 examination, she asked if we had any data questions that she could use for practice. 'One or two' might have been the initial reply. Instead, however, we started writing down our collection, many of which are real-life scenarios, actually seen and managed in our hospital. These questions started life in a simple format of blocks of 10. Inevitably, however, with our usual desire to explore the limits of opportunity, this very rapidly evolved into a major project, culminating in what you see before you - our personal, but definitive, guide to answering MRCPCH data questions.

2001   J.L.R.
                                                                     A.P.H.

Contents

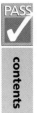

contents

Introduction

Answering any exam question is a mixture of knowledge and technique. In our experience, the best technique for answering data questions is as follows:

1. Firstly highlight those parts of the question which you believe are relevant.
2. Then read *all* the stems of the question, *before* attempting to answer it.
3. Having answered the question, see if the answers are appropriate for all the highlighted part.
4. If not, think again – it may be that the answer is wrong; or
5. It may be that certain things underlined are not relevant.

For instance, beware the haematological question with 'Greek child' in it. Thalassaemia may be the correct association, but some Greek children will be iron deficient. The information *may* or *may not* be relevant.

The following example demonstrates the usefulness of this answering system (the italicized words are those you will have highlighted):

A 10-day-old female infant presents to you with *vomiting* and *drowsiness*. On examination she is *dehydrated* and has *normal genitalia*.

Sodium	118 mmol/L
Urea	20.8 mmol/L
Glucose	1.8 mmol/L

(a) What is the cause of this child's presenting illness?
(b) What is the underlying diagnosis?

You may answer that the child has a salt-losing crisis and congenital adrenal hyperplasia. This may well be right. However, the question specifically says that the baby has *normal* genitalia and therefore the better answer is that of congenital adrenal hypoplasia.

HOW TO USE THIS BOOK

This book is designed to explain *how* to answer the questions, as opposed to explaining the answers. Most of the chapters are divided into five sections:

- Questions (1).
- Answers to questions (1) with brief explanations where relevant.
- Helpful hints. This may need reading several times but will help get you to the answers.

You should now be in a position to answer the second set of questions more appropriately and improve your performance in doing so.

- Questions (2).
- Answers to questions (2).

The book finishes with three exams that should be completed under exam conditions with appropriate time limits.

Respiratory medicine

QUESTIONS (1)

1.1 You are asked to review the lung function tests on a nine-year-old boy.

	Predicted	Measured	
FVC	2.06	1.30	(63%)
FEV$_1$	1.86	1.05	(51%)
PEF	272	212	

(a) What type of picture do these results demonstrate?

(b) Give the two most likely underlying conditions.

√1.2 A six-year-old boy is reviewed in your respiratory clinic. He is known to have cystic fibrosis.

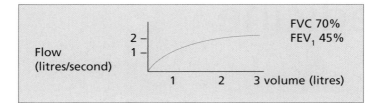

(a) What do the results suggest?

_____

(b) What is an appropriate follow up test?

_____

1.3 A 16-year-old girl has had well-controlled asthma for the past two years. When reviewed in clinic this time, the following test results were found.

	Predicted	Measured
FVC (litres)	3.97	3.02
FEV$_1$ (litres)	3.82	1.72
FEF (25–75%)	4.05	1.08

Suggest two possible explanations.

_____

_____

1.4 The following lung function tests were obtained from a 10-year-old boy with cystic fibrosis before and after a one-month course of treatment.

	Predicted	Measured	1 month later
FVC	2.1	1.21 (57%)	1.59 (76%)
FEV$_1$	1.90	1.00 (53%)	1.25 (65%)
PEF	277	205	197

(a) What is the likely treatment?

(b) What is the percentage rise in FEV$_1$?

1.5 These are the lung function tests of a 15-year-old asthmatic with exercise intolerance.

	Predicted	Measured
FVC	3.91	3.68
FEV$_1$	3.75	2.96
PEF	471	425

She is on moderate doses of inhaled steroids. Give two possible treatment options.

1.6 Below is a diagram of lung volumes.

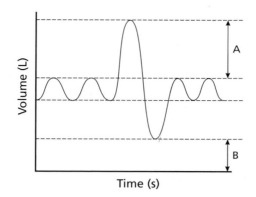

(a) What do the letters A and B represent?

_____

_____

(b) Mark the vital capacity (as C) and expiratory reserve volume (as D) on the diagram.

1.1 (a) Restrictive lung disease.

(b) A neuromuscular condition (such as muscular dystrophy).

Comment: Both FVC and FEV_1 are markedly reduced. This may also occur in fibrosing alveolitis or fibrosis from other conditions, and in kyphoscoliosis. Note that cystic fibrosis is usually mixed.

1.2 (a) Restrictive and obstructive lung disease.

(b) Repeat after bronchodilators to see if there is a reversible component.

Comment: FVC is reduced but FEV_1 is reduced by a lot more.

1.3 Poor compliance, smoking or a worsening of her asthma.

The GP had in fact reduced the dose as the patient was well controlled.

Comment: Always put the most likely answer first.

1.4 (a) DNase

(b) 25%

Comment: $\dfrac{1.25 \times 1.00}{1.00} \times 100 = 25\%$

1.5 Add an inhaled long-acting beta-agonist, increase the inhaled steroids, or give oral anti-leukotrienes.

Comment: Asthma guidelines.

You do not need to name specific drugs.

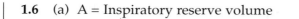
1.6 (a) A = Inspiratory reserve volume

B = Residual lung volume

(b)

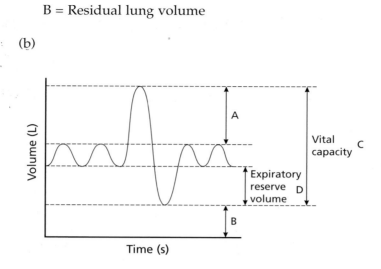

Comment: Remember that one division is always a volume and more than one is always a capacity.

Helpful hints

LUNG FUNCTION TESTS

1. FVC + FEV$_1$: if both are low this suggests a restrictive picture. $\frac{FEV_1}{FVC}$ N = 7S-80%. or high

2. FVC near normal with low FEV$_1$ suggests obstructive picture. $\frac{FEV_1}{FVC}$ ⌄40%.

3. FVC low, but FEV$_1$ a lot lower suggests a mixed picture.

For example

	Predicted	Result (1)	Result (2)	Result (3)
FVC	2.00	1.30↓	1.8→	1.5↓
FEV$_1$	1.86	1.05↓	1.2↓	1.05↓↓
		Restricted	Obstructive	Mixed

4. This may be expressed as a graph with only the percentage of predictive for FVC and FEV$_1$.

5. The most common restrictive pattern in children is muscular dystrophy and severe scoliosis.

6. The most common obstructive pattern is asthma.

7. CF may be shown as a purely restrictive set of results but is often mixed.

QUESTIONS (2)

1.7 Draw a diagram of lung volumes showing the following:

A = Vital capacity

B = Functional residual capacity

C = Tidal volume

D = Expiratory reserve volume

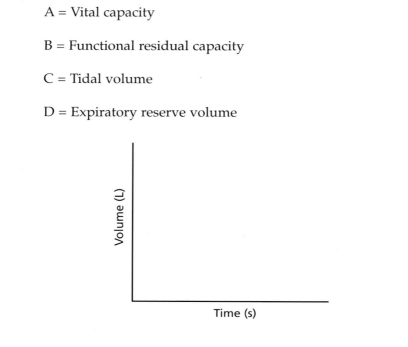

1.8 For the past two winters, a three-year-old child had been noted to suffer from lethargy and coughing which seems to settle each spring. This has been associated with poor feeding. The house is old but not damp and has no central heating. The local authority intervened three weeks ago and the child is now much better.

(a) What is the diagnosis?

(b) What has the council done?

1.9 A 16-year-old boy has been followed up in your clinic for several years. These are his latest lung function tests.

	Predicted	Measured	%
FVC	4.04	3.50	85
FEV$_1$	3.88	2.21	57
PEF	481	253	53
FEF (25–75%)	4.09	1.70	41

(a) What is the diagnosis?

(b) Which of the above measurements is best for monitoring his condition?

1.10 The following results were found when reviewing a 15-year-old asthmatic. She is on inhaled steroids (800 µg b.d.) and a long-acting beta 2 agonist (2 puffs b.d.)

	Predicted	Measured	%
FVC	3.97	4.51	114
FEV$_1$	3.82	3.75	98
PEF	476	491	103
FEF (25–75%)	4.05	3.76	93

What is your management plan?

1.11 This seven-year-old has cystic fibrosis and poor exercise tolerance. These are his lung function tests.

FVC	83%	predicted
FEV$_1$	50%	predicted
FEF (25–75%)	50%	predicted

(a) What test would you do next?

(b) What treatment would you try?

1.7

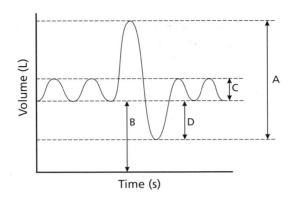

Comment: Remember one space is a volume.

1.8 (a) Carbon monoxide poisoning.

(b) Changed the gas heating.

Comment: Nothing else fits all the relevant parts – for example, asthma would not usually cause poor feeding.

1.9 (a) Asthma.

(b) FEF (25–75%).

Comment: FEF (25–75%) is the best measurement of small airway disease. Peak flows are used because of their ease in measurement but they mainly reflect large airways.

1.10 Decrease the inhaled steroids.

Comment: 800 µg b.d. is a high dose and the results showed control.

1.11 (a) Bronchodilator response.

(b) Bronchodilators/inhaled steroids/oral steroids.

Comment: FEV_1 and FEF (25–75%) are markedly reduced suggesting airway obstruction. If there is a bronchodilator response, treatment with bronchodilators plus inhaler or oral steroids may not help.

Cardiology

QUESTIONS (1)

2.1 The following are cardiac catheter results in a non-cyanotic 18-month-old child.

	Saturation (%)	Pressure (mmHg)
SVC	79	
RA	88	
RV	86	
PA	86	
LA	96	– / 6
LV	96	
A	96	

(a) What is the underlying diagnosis?

(b) What pressure would you expect in the right atrium?

(2.2) These cardiac catheterization results were obtained on a four-month-old premature baby.

	Saturation (%)
RA	50
RV	50
PA	50
LA	80
LV	80
A	86

(a) Give the most likely diagnosis.

(b) What further information do you need to confirm?

2.3 Match the three groups of cardiac lesions to the three syndromes:– Trisomy 13, 18 and 21.

(a) PDA, septal defects, pulmonary, aortic stenosis.

(b) AVSD, VSD, PDA.

(c) VSD, polyvalvular disease, coronary abnormalities

2.4 A three-year-old has a cardiac catheterization.

	Saturation (%)	BP
RA	74	–/3
RV	74	70/30
PA	74	25/10
LA	96	
LV	96	

(a) What is the diagnosis?

(b) Name two changes that may occur on the ECG.

2.5 You are asked to see a six-year-old boy who has seen his GP for headaches. His blood pressure is 150/70. You notice he has a murmur.

(a) What is the most likely diagnosis?

(b) Draw a table of approximate pressures and saturations for the left side.

	Saturations	Pressures
LA	96	– / 10
LV		
Ascending aorta		
Descending aorta		

2.1 (a) Atrial septal defect.

(b) −/6.

Comment: Saturations are too high in the right atrium so this is the level of the shunt.

2.2 (a) Chronic lung disease.

(b) Echocardiogram.

Comment: Chronic lung disease is the diagnosis because you would not get Eisenmenger through an atrial septal defect by 4 months.

2.3 (a) 18,

(b) 21,

(c) 13.

2.4 (a) Pulmonary stenosis.

(b) Right ventricular hypertrophy – upright T-wave V_1

Tall R-wave V_1

Right axis deviation.

Comment: The saturations are appropriate so it must be a valve problem, therefore look at the pressures.

2.5 (a) Aortic coarctation.

(b)

	Saturations	Pressures
LA	96	–/10
LV	96	150/70
Ascending aorta	96	150/70
Descending abdominal aorta	96	70/30

Comment: An acyanotic lesion, so there is no drop in saturations. The pressures do not have to be precise but there is already one in the question.

Clue to answer (b): include ascending and descending.

Helpful hints

INTERPRETATION OF CARDIAC CATHETERIZATION

Draw a schematic heart. For example:

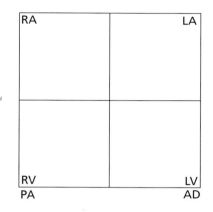

RA	LA
RV	LV
PA	AD

1. Mark the saturations in the boxes.

  (a) Ask:

      Are the saturations on the left greater than 90? Yes = normal.

      Are the saturations on the right less than 80? Yes = normal.

      Are they staying the same as the blood passes from one chamber to the next?

  (b) A step up on the right indicates a left to right shunt.

  (c) A step down on the left indicates a right to left shunt.

2. Now mark all the blood pressures in the boxes.

    (a) All the right sides should be lower than the left.

    (b) If they are equal at any level then there may be shunting.

    (c) If there is a step down across a valve then it is suggestive of stenosis.

    (d) This is especially true if you see a higher than expected pressure in the chamber before the step down; for example, in pulmonary stenosis this would be in the right ventricle.

Examples

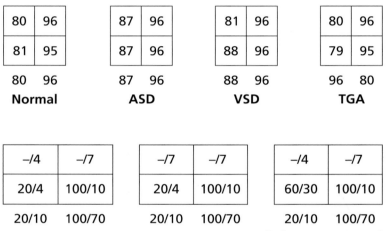

2.6 You are reviewing a two-year-old with the following cardiac pressures.

He is acyanotic.

	Pressure (mmHg)
RA	–/3
RV	50/20
Pulmonary	50/20
LA	–/7
LV	100/70
Aorta	100/70

(a) What is the diagnosis?

(b) What saturations would you expect in:

    (i) RA?

    (ii) RV?

2.7 You see a three-week-old baby whom you suspect has cyanotic heart disease. These are the cardiac catheterization results.

	Saturation (%)
RA	80
RV	80
Pulmonary	95
LA	95
LV	95
Aortic	80

(a) Are you right?

(b) What is the correct diagnosis?

2.8 A five-year-old child is seen by the cardiologist having been referred for a murmur that radiates to his back.

Cardiac catheterization shows:

	Pressure (mmHg)	Saturation (%)
RV	41/6	80
Left pulmonary	25/15	89
Aorta	98/53	99

(a) What is the diagnosis?

_____

(b) What is the treatment of choice?

_____

2.9 These are the cardiac catheterisation pressures of a 13-year-old pre- and post intervention.

	Pre-Intervention	Post intervention
Left ventricle	155/30	139/23
Ascending aorta	95/7	98/54
Descending aorta	109/63	

(a) What is the diagnosis?

(b) Give two ways he may have presented.

2.6 (a) Ventricular septal defect (could be patent ductus arteriosus (PDA) but part (b) suggests VSD).

(b) (i) 80 (ii) 86

Comment: The pressure is increased in the right ventricle so in (b) show a step up here.

2.7 (a) Yes.

(b) Transposition of the great arteries.

Comment: Be careful, at first glance the saturations look normal.

2.8 (a) PDA.

(b) Closed coil or plug.

Comment: The increase in both saturations and pressure shows a left to right shunt.

2.9 (a) Aortic stenosis.

(b) Incidental murmur or collapse.

Comment: This is caused by a drop in blood pressure across the valve.

ECGs

3

QUESTIONS (1)

3.1 Comment on the axis of this ECG.

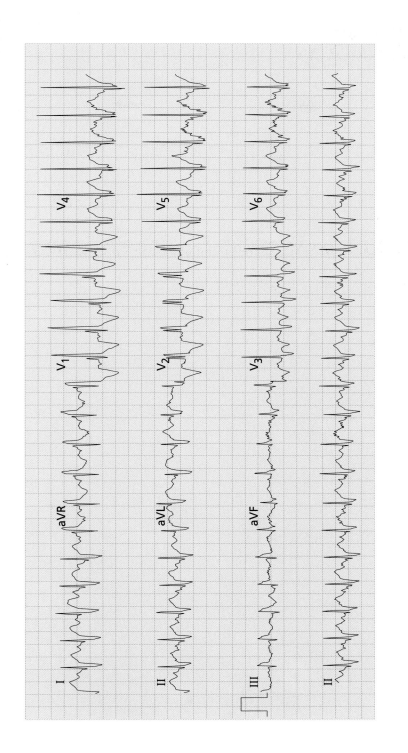

3.2 This is the ECG of a 14-year-old girl who had a fontan operation for tricuspid atresia and pulmonary stenosis. Comment on the right atrium and ventricle.

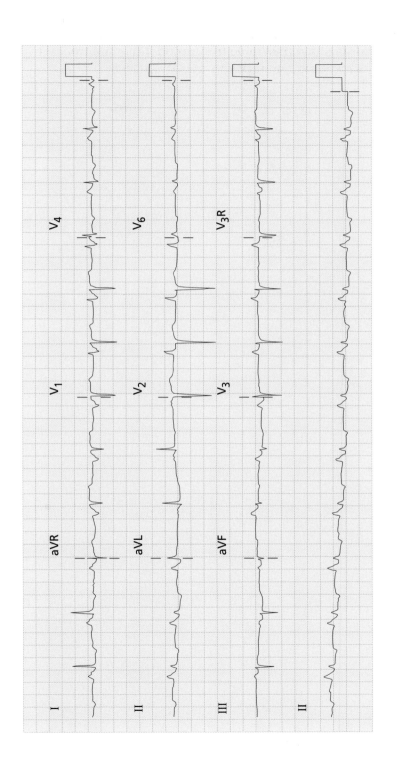

3.3 This is an ECG of a five-year-old girl who was operated on for transposition. List three features on it that indicate right ventricular hypertrophy.

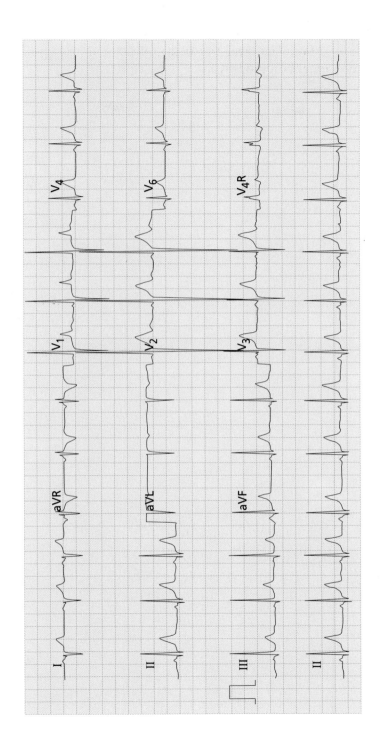

3.4 This 20-day-old baby with Down syndrome has cyanosis.

(a) Comment on the ECG.

_____

_____

(b) What is the cause of the cyanosis?

_____

_____

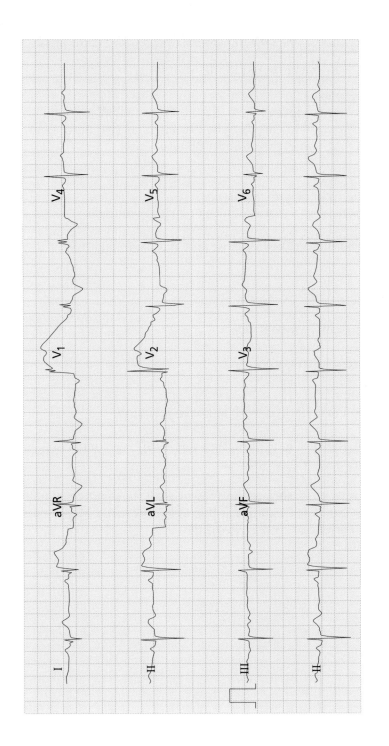

3.1   You cannot comment on the axis as there is a wide QRS complex.

Comment: This needs to be explained as two lines. Look at V_1 – M-wave, therefore RBBB (see hints).

3.2   The right atrium is enlarged.
There is minimal evidence of a right ventricle.

Comment: Peaked P-wave and V_3R is all negative.

3.3   Right axis

Upright T-wave V_1 V_2

Peaked R-wave V_1.

3.4   (a) Partial R BBB with left axis deviation.

(b) Right to left shunt, through AVSD – secondary to pulmonary hypertension.

Comment: Associate the answer with the syndrome! It is not Eisenmenger, because at this age it is caused by pulmonary hypertension and is reversible.

Helpful hints

HOW TO READ AN ECG

1. Look at the rhythm strip for:

(a) Rate

(b) Rhythm

(c) Is there a P wave for each QRS?

2. Look at the leads V_1–V_6 to see where V_4R is. Look at the standardization mark to check millivoltage.

3. Look at the axis:
either

(a) I and aVF.

Work out the number of positive or negative squares and then plot the axis.

For example

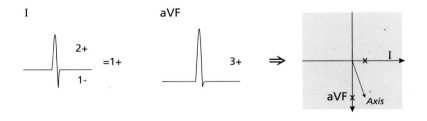

or

(b) The axis is at right angles to the smallest most equiphasic lead. Then look at the lead at right angles; if it is positive the axis is towards it.

For example, if the equiphasic lead is aVf look at lead I.

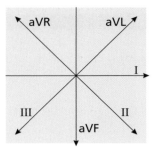

4. Look for bundle branch block (BBB). This is usually right BBB with M in V_1. Left BBB is exceptionally uncommon both in child and paediatric exams (largely because it is not associated with congenital heart disease).

Pneumonic: Marrow and William

M   M in lead V_1

A

R   R for right

R

O

W   W in lead V_6

W   W in lead V_1

I

L   L for left

L

I

A

M   M in lead V_6

NB

(a) Complete BBB (that is, wide QRS complex) means you cannot comment on the axis.

(b) Partial BBB (that is, normal width QRS complex) means you can comment on the axis.

(c) RBBB means you cannot comment on right ventricular hypertrophy.

5. Look for atrial hypertrophy in leads II, V_1.

(a) P-wave too tall = right atrium

(b) P-wave bifid = left atrium

6. Remember age dominance:

For example, at birth right ventricle

Then mixed dominance

Progressing to left ventricle

(a)	Right ventricle dominant	Mainly R-wave V_1
		Mainly S-wave V_6
(b)	Left ventricle dominant	Mainly S-wave V_1
		Mainly R-wave V_6

Dominance usually changes from right to <u>left in the first months.</u>

7. Look for ventricular hypertrophy:

(a) Right ventricular hypertrophy

✓R-wave > 20 mm V_1

S-wave > 5 mm V_6

Right axis deviation

Positive T-wave V_1

(b) Left ventricular hypertrophy

S-wave > 20 mm V_1

R-wave > 25 mm V_6

(c) Combined is a mixture of the above.

8. Look for a delta wave. This must be associated with a short P–R interval. (P–R is from start of P-wave till start of QRS complex. Normal 0.12 ms = 3 squares.) It may help to place a piece of paper along the R-wave.

NB This may be mistaken for BBB.

9. The T-wave should be negative from day 7 till 12 years in V_1.

10. $K^+ \downarrow$ = Flat T   or = Ca $\uparrow$

$K^+ \uparrow$ = peaked T   or = Ca $\downarrow$

Now you have read the ECG, read the question and fit it together.

For example

(a) Partial RBBB   = ASD

then <u>R</u>ight axis = Secundum

Left axis   = P<u>r</u>imum

(Remember one R in each)

(b) Left ventricular hypertrophy

Think coarctation and aortic stenosis, for example.

3.5 This is the ECG of a 12-year-old girl who had a fontans procedure for tricuspid atresia. There is no murmur and BP is 85/50.

What does the ECG show?

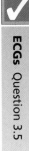
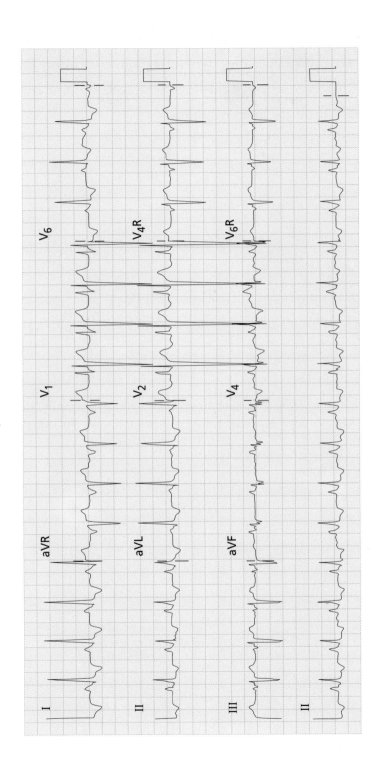

PASS ✓

3.6 You have seen a three-month-old baby with the cardiologist. The baby has poor weight gain and feeding difficulty. The echocardiogram shows significant pulmonary artery branch stenosis.

(a) What is the likely diagnosis?

(b) How is this confirmed?

(c) What other blood test needs checking?

3.7 This is an ECG of a 16-year-old boy who is normally asymptomatic but was noted to have ectopics during surgery.

(a) What does the ECG show?

(b) Is he likely to need an operation?

(c) How might you confirm that they are benign?

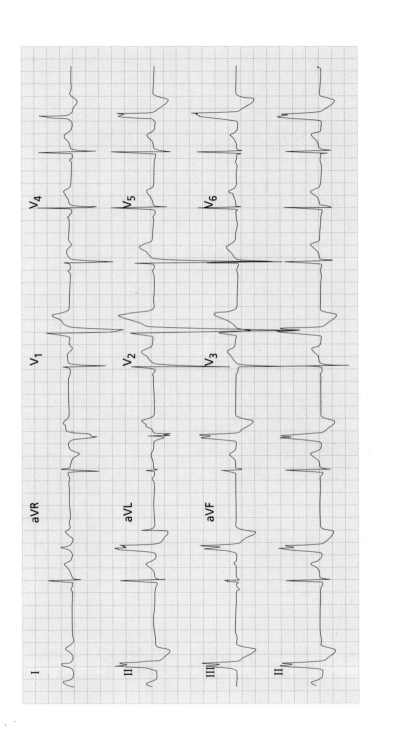

PASS ✓

3.8 You are reviewing a five-month-old baby with known pulmonary artery branch stenosis with the following ECG.

What features are notable on the ECG?

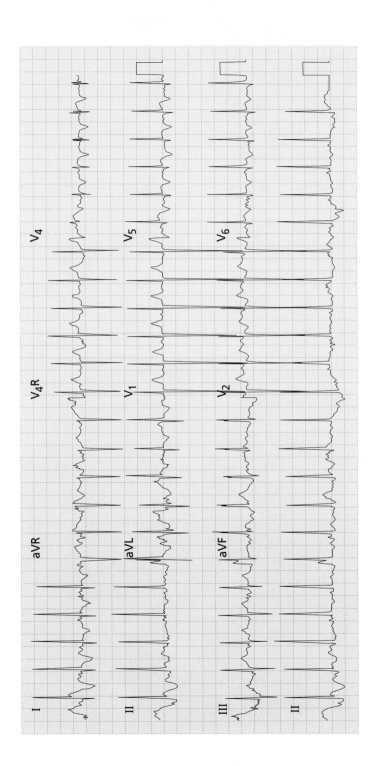

I   aVR   V₄R   V₄

II   aVL   V₁   V₅

III   aVF   V₂   V₆

II

3.5 Right atrial hypertrophy.

Left axis deviation.

3.6 (a) Williams syndrome.

(b) FISH test: deletion long arm chromosome 7.

(c) Calcium can be hypercalcaemic.

Comment: You can use initials but where possible write in full.

3.7 (a) Bigemini with unifocal ventricular ectopics.

(b) No.

(c) They disappear with exercise.

Comment: Asymptomatic and normal complex in between.

3.8 Upright T- wave V_1

Inverted T-wave V_6

Comment: Look for the clue in the question – for example, pulmonary stenosis therefore look at the right ventricle.

Audiometry

4.1 You are asked to see a five-year-old boy whose mother is worried that he watches television with the volume turned up too loud.

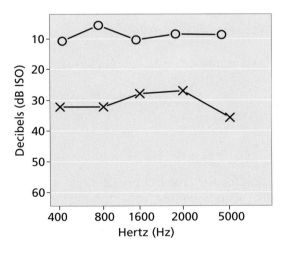

What is the diagnosis?

4.2 You are asked to review the following Rinne and Weber results.

Right   Rinne   positive

Left   Rinne   negative

Weber   to the left

What would you expect the audiogram to show?

_____

_____

4.3 You are shown the following audiogram of a six-year-old who has a complication of a childhood illness.

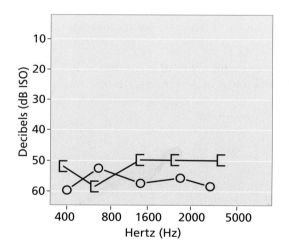

(a) What does it show?

_____

(b) Name a possible childhood illness

_____

4.4 A four-year-old boy is tired during the day and dribbling a lot. He is developmentally normal.

(a) What two questions would you ask?

(b) Name two tests to confirm the diagnosis

4.5 A child has sensorineural deafness on the left. What would be the results from Rinne and Weber tests?

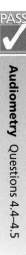

4.6 These are the tympanogram results from a three-year-old boy.

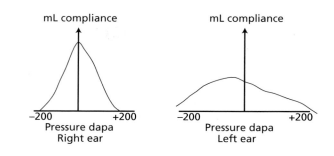

What diagnosis does it suggest?

_____

4.1 Left conductive hearing loss.

Comments: Always make sure you indicate which ear. The hearing loss is less than 40 decibels, so is conductive.

4.2 Left conductive hearing loss.

Normal right ear.

Comments: The ear that is Rinne negative is always the abnormal one.

4.3 (a) Right sensorineural loss.

(b) Mumps or meningitis.

4.4 (a) Does he snore?

Does he have pauses in his snoring?

(b) Overnight saturations.

Arterial blood gas while asleep.

Comments: Diagnosis is usually made on history.

4.5 Rinne – left negative

right positive

Weber to the right

4.6 Acute otitis media on the left.

Comments: Left tympanogram flattened and shifted to the left.

Helpful hints

AUDIOMETRY

1. Which ear? This is easily remembered by Right O (chaps), and therefore X is left.

2. Normal hearing is from 0 → −20.

3. Conductive hearing loss from −20 → −40.

4. Sensorineural loss is from −40 +.

5. If the examiners give you a conductive hearing loss of greater than −40 then they will also give bone conduction, which will be a lot better.

6. If the examiners give you a sensorineural hearing loss of less than −40 then they will show bone conduction at a similar level.

Examples

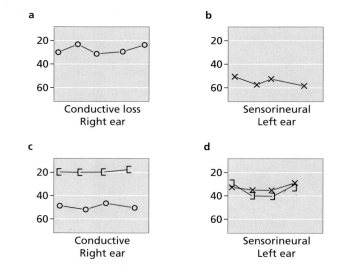

a — Conductive loss / Right ear

b — Sensorineural / Left ear

c — Conductive / Right ear

d — Sensorineural / Left ear

The Rinne test compares air and bone conduction for one ear, and is performed by putting the tuning fork near the ear until it cannot be heard, then putting it on the mastoid process. If it is audible again then it is Rinne negative.

The Weber test compares the bone conduction of both ears. It is placed in the centre of the forehead.

1. The ear that is Rinne negative is *always* the abnormal one.

2. If the Weber test is towards the abnormal ears it is conductive hearing loss.

3. If the Weber test is away from that ear it is sensorineural hearing loss.

4. If both Rinne tests are negative then:

   (a) Weber central means that both ears have either sensorineural or conductive loss.

   (b) Weber towards one ear means that ear has conductive loss and the other ear sensorineural loss.

4.7 This is the audiogram of a five-year-old girl.

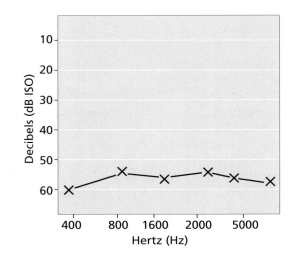

(a) Which ear is it?

_____

(b) Add (i) Bone conduction for *sensorineural* deafness.

(ii) Bone conduction for *conductive* deafness.

4.8 These are the tympanograms of a two-year-old boy.

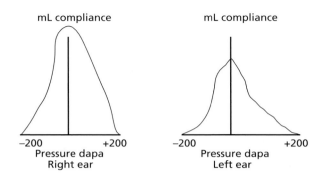

mL compliance

mL compliance

−200   +200
Pressure dapa
Right ear

−200   +200
Pressure dapa
Left ear

If the left ear is normal, what would you expect to see in the right ear on examination?

4.9 This is the hearing test of a six-year-old boy with Down syndrome.

Right   Rinne negative

Left   Rinne negative

Weber   central

(a) What is the differential diagnosis?

(b) Which diagnosis is more likely?

4.10 This is an audiogram of a three-year-old referred to an ENT surgeon.

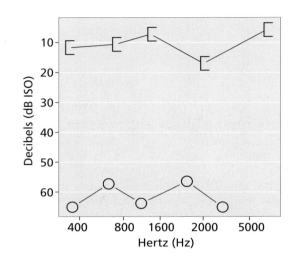

(a) What does it show?

_____

(b) Does he need an operation?

_____

4.7 (a) The left ear.

(b)

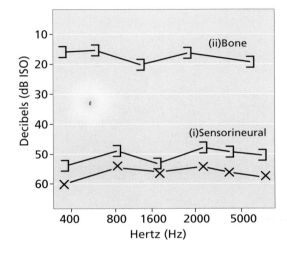

4.8 The right ear may be normal, but may have a thin ear drum (hyper mobile) or ossicular discontinuity.

4.9 (a) Bilateral conductive or sensorineural hearing loss.

(b) Conductive.

Comment: Conductive hearing loss is more common in Down syndrome babies, but also in any child with a facial problem such as cleft palate or snoring.

4.10 (a) Severe conductive hearing loss of right ear.

(b) Yes.

Neurology

5

5.1 A 13-year-old boy is admitted with his second generalized tonic–clonic seizure, but on closer questioning is said to be quite 'jumpy' in the mornings, such that he tends to spill drinks at breakfast and drop his pen at school. The EEG findings are shown on the opposite page.

(a) Describe the EEG findings.

(b) What is the diagnosis?

5.2 At <u>six days</u> old, a baby girl developed myoclonic and tonic seizures, unresponsive to standard anti-epilepsy drugs. Daily seizures continued unabated, and the EEG at four weeks of age is shown.

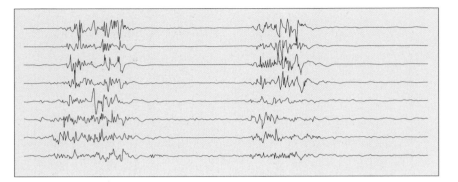

(a) Describe the EEG pattern.

(b) Suggest a likely diagnosis.

5.3 A <u>seven-year-old</u> girl was referred because of concerns about lapses in concentration and deterioration in school work.

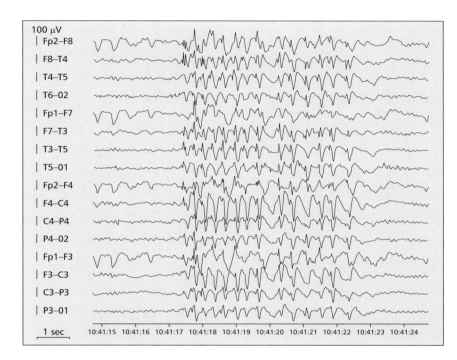

(a) What does the EEG demonstrate?

(b) What practical manoeuvre may help with the diagnosis in clinic?

(c) What is the diagnosis?

5.4 An eight-month-old infant, admitted with crying episodes, is noted to have intermittent abnormal movements causing distress.

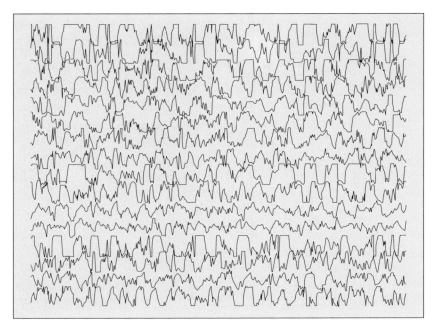

(a) What does his EEG show?

(b) What is the diagnosis?

5.5 An 11-year-old girl presented with a three-month history of episodic staring lasting <u>two</u> minutes, accompanied by excessive swallowing and occasional inappropriate laughter.

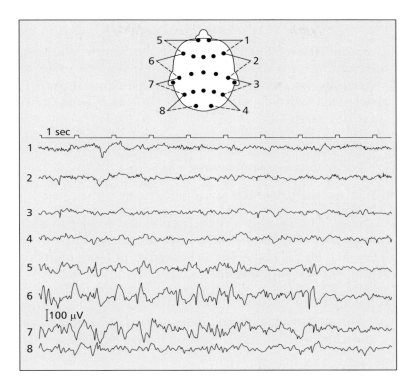

(a) Describe the EEG findings.

(b) What is the diagnosis?

(c) What is the most appropriate next investigation?

5.1 (a) Generalized irregular spike-wave complex.

(b) Juvenile myoclonic epilepsy.

Comment: History and age are important: 'jumpy' with spills in the morning (or when tired) = myoclonic seizures; often presents as first/second generalized tonic–clonic seizure; EEG generalized (across whole montage) with short-lived spike-wave discharge.

5.2 (a) Burst suppression pattern.

(b) Severe early neonatal myoclonic epilepsy.

Comment: History, age, very early onset and progressive (malignant). EEG shows bursts of abnormal chaotic activity on a very flat virtually iso-electric background – very ominous and typical of burst suppression.

5.3 (a) Abrupt onset generalized 3 per second spike and wave discharges.

(b) Hyperventilation.

(c) Childhood onset typical of absence epilepsy.

Comment – The history may not make specific reference to absences.

– Watch out for the same question with normal EEG (the diagnosis may then be attentional/learning difficulties).

– Age is important for precise diagnosis (childhood onset, juvenile onset etc.)

– Do not use the term petit mal.

– Slower frequency may indicate atypical absence epilepsy.

– Beware hyperventilation indicator on montage.

This is a blueprint (diagnostic) EEG.

5.4 (a) Hypsarrhythmia.

(b) Infantile spasms.

Comment: History: a common presentation masquerading as colic. It could be West syndrome, but there is no specific mention of developmental delay at presentation. The underlying diagnosis (for example tuberous sclerosis) cannot be determined by EEG alone. Blueprint EEG diagnostic when present – chaotic disorganized background with multi-focal high amplitude spikes and slow waves.

5.5 (a) Spike discharges in the left temporal area.

(b) Complex partial seizures.

(c) MRI of the brain.

Comment: History: episodes too long for typical absence, and associated with unusual mannerisms, suggest complex partial seizures (formerly known as temporal lobe epilepsy). EEG: focal spike-discharges in leads 6 and 7 (left temporal region). MRI is now the first-choice investigation for looking at temporal lobes in detail.

Helpful hints

THE EEG

1. Read the history carefully as this can give the diagnosis before looking at the EEG.

2. EEG abnormalities are likely to be obvious or 'blueprint'/diagnostic.

3. Montage (that is, orientation of leads):

- Left is left and right is right as you look at the montage.

- Labelling may vary but should always allow you to match up the labels on the montage with the corresponding leads on the EEG (and hence identify relevant area of the brain).

- Ignore the montage if the abnormality is apparent across all leads (that is, generalized).

- ✔ If there is no montage in the exam the EEG is very likely to show a generalized abnormality.

4. **Basic principles:**

- Is the abnormality across all leads ? If so this is a generalized epilepsy.

- Is the abnormality across the leads of one side/one or two leads only? If so this is a partial/focal epilepsy.

- Is the abnormality paroxysmal, for example spike-wave discharges/spike discharges?

- Is the abnormality periodic, for example burst suppression or SSPE?

- Is the abnormality continuous, for example hypsarrhythmia or status epilepticus?

- Is the abnormality rhythmic or disorganized/chaotic?

5. **Look for:**

(a) Second (time-scale) marker to identify frequency (for instance 3 per second spike-wave discharge).

(b) Photic stimulation marker – may precede photo-paroxysmal response.

(c) Hyperventilation marker – may precede 3 per second spike-wave discharges.

(d) ECG trace (at the bottom of the EEG recording). This may identify alternative (for example cardiac) cause for collapse.

5.6 A 14-year-old girl with moderate learning difficulties and myoclonic epilepsy presented with a 24 h history of unresponsiveness, staring and fumbling with her clothes. The EEG shown is representative of the whole 20 min EEG recording.

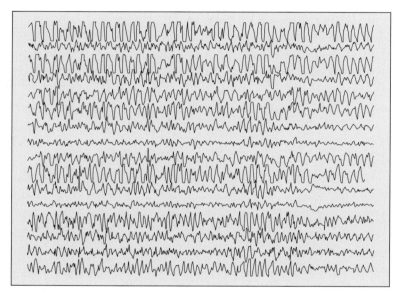

(a) What is the diagnosis?

_____

(b) What would be your immediate management?

_____

_____

5.7 A 10-year-old boy, initially referred to the child psychiatrist with a behavioural disorder, has shown a progressive deterioration in written work over the last six months at school. More recently he has fallen over a number of times, appearing to lose his balance.

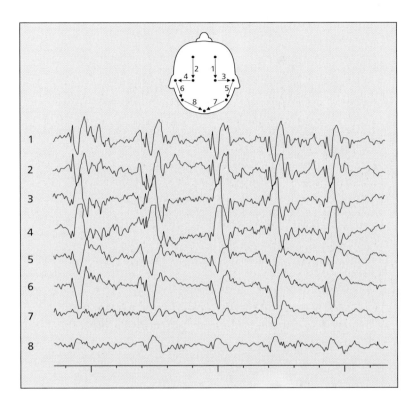

(a) What does his EEG show?

(b) What is the diagnosis?

5.8 An eight-year-old boy presents in the early hours of the morning, following his first generalized tonic-clonic seizure. On closer questioning, it is found that he has experienced frequent episodes of unilateral facial paraesthesia for four months, followed by choking sensations and twitching of the lips and cheek. These occur on awakening, and he is unable to communicate during such episodes.

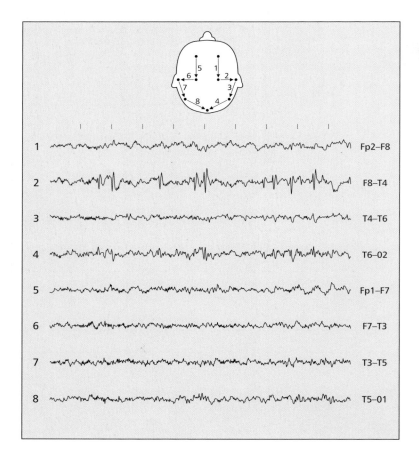

(a) What does his EEG demonstrate?

(b) What is the diagnosis?

5.9 A seven-year-old boy with severe learning difficulties was diagnosed with West syndrome at six months of age, and continues to experience frequent multiple seizure types (including tonic, atonic and myoclonic seizures).

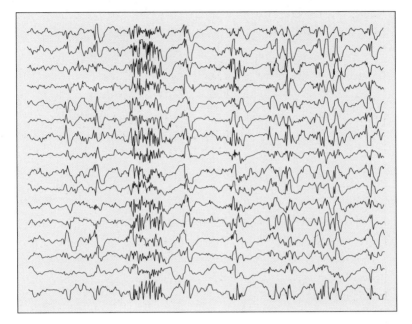

(a) Describe his EEG.

_____

(b) What is the diagnosis?

_____

5.10 A teenage boy has juvenile myoclonic epilepsy.

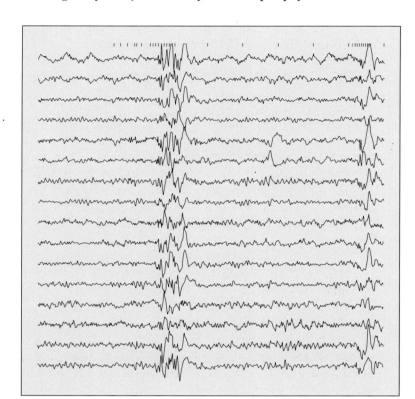

(a) What does the EEG show?

_____

(b) What might the technician have witnessed during this period of the recording?

_____

5.6　(a)　Complex partial status epilepticus.

(b)　Intravenous bolus of diazepam.

Comment: The history is very suggestive of complex partial/atypical absence/non-convulsive status epilepticus. (EEG shows a virtually continuous slow wave activity across all leads, and throughout the whole of the recording.) Treatment is with intravenous benzodiazepine rather than rectal (because of 24 h history). May need infusion; this is often undertaken 'under EEG control', but this is not essential and will usually see patient 'wake up' following/during administration.

5.7　(a)　Large-amplitude periodic slow wave complexes, occurring every 3.5–4 s.

(b)　Sub-acute sclerosing panencephalitis.

Comment: Look at the history and age (in fact 10 years is quite young for SSPE). Patients are often referred as having behavioural/psychiatric problems. There is progressive neurological regression including ataxia. EEG shows typical periodic appearance across all leads.

5.8　(a)　Unilateral right-sided centro-temporal spike-waves.

(b)　Benign Rolandic epilepsy of childhood.

Comment: The history and age are important. Typical presentation in early hours of the morning (usually during sleep); typical history of partial sensory motor seizures (involving face, plus or minus upper limb). Beware as this often presents as apparent first generalized tonic–clonic seizure (but is a partial epilepsy). Alternative label/diagnosis is 'benign partial epilepsy of childhood with centro-temporal (Rolandic) spikes'. Blueprint EEG and diagnostic.

5.9 (a) Generalized multiple discharges of spike-wave and poly-spike complexes.

(b) Lennox–Gastaut syndrome.

Comment: History.(Important cause of developmental arrest – intractable multiple seizure types are often resistant to standard anti-epileptic drugs. Age at presentation is important. Previous history of West syndrome is common. EEG is not as chaotic as hypsarrhythmia: multiple spike and poly-spikes are typical.)

5.10 (a) Generalized spike wave discharge secondary to photic stimulation.

(b) Myoclonic jerk.

Comment: Look at the EEG photic stimulation 'markers'. It would be reasonable to suggest myoclonic jerk, absence or eyelid flickering as a clinical (photo-convulsive) response. May have similar EEG photo-paroxysmal response *without* any clinical change.

Genetics

QUESTIONS (1)

6.1 You are seeing patients (a) and (b) below who show you the following family tree:

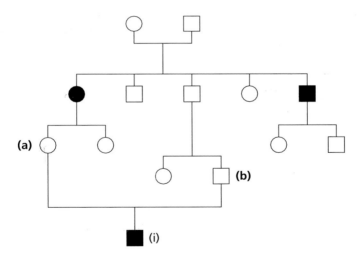

(a) What is the mode of inheritance?

_____

(b) If you were seeing (a) and (b) antenatally, what is the chance of (a) having the condition?

_____

6.2 The following family history has been worked out:

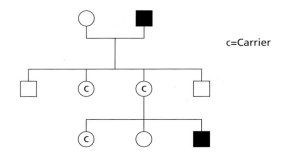

c=Carrier

What is the mode of inheritance?

_____

6.3 A baby is born with a cleft palate and found to have a heart murmur. This is shown to be tetralogy of Fallot.

(a) What is the likely diagnosis?

_____

(b) Name a confirmatory test.

_____

6.4

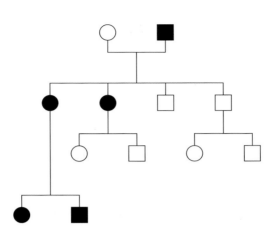

What is the mode of inheritance?

_____

6.5 The karyotype is 46 xy −14 + t (14q 21q)

(a) Describe the above.

_____

(b) What are the recurrence risks?

_____

_____

_____

6.6 A girl is admitted, drowsy, having had a history of a viral illness.

There is a family history of SIDS and her mother has an increased orotic acid.

(a) What is the likely diagnosis?

_____

(b) What is its mode of inheritance?

_____

(c) How will you confirm the diagnosis?

_____

6.1 (a) Autosomal recessive

(b) $\frac{2}{3} \times \frac{1}{2} \times 1 \times \frac{1}{4} = \frac{1}{12}$

Comment:

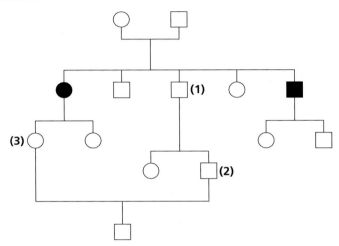

Look at one generation at a time.

For example (1) =

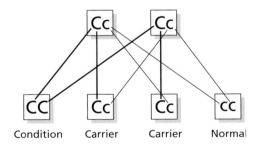

| Condition | Carrier | Carrier | Normal |

As we already know that (1) has not got the condition $\frac{2}{3}$ are carriers.

Then (2) = $\frac{1}{2}$ because we assume that (1) marries a non-carrier. (3) Again, assuming that the father is a non-carrier then the mother must pass the affected gene on.

PASS ✓

6.2 X-linked recessive.

Comment: The father passes it to all his daughters, but they are only carriers, and none of his sons. The mother can make daughters carriers and affect sons.

6.3 (a) DiGeorge syndrome.

(b) FISH assay looking at chromosome 15.

Comment: This is an example of best fitting a syndrome to a set of clinical features.

6.4 X-linked dominant.

Comment: Always look to see who can inherit from whom. It could be autosomal dominant but the tree shows two sons not getting it from their father.

6.5 (a) Male unbalanced Robertsonian 14, 21 translocation.

(b) Neither parent is a carrier: 1%; mother carrier: 10%; father carrier: 2.3%.

Comment: Do not forget to mention the sex of the fetus. In the second part there are three lines looking for three answers. Remember to provide as many answers as there are lines for doing so on the question paper.

6.6 (a) Ornithine Carbamyl Transferase deficiency.

(b) X-linked recessive.

(c) Urinary orotic acid levels.

Helpful hints

1. Autosomal dominant + recessive can go from mother and father to sons and daughters.

2. Autosomal recessive usually results from relations marrying.

3. X-linked recessive: mothers can only give it to sons and daughters have 50/50 chance of carriage.

4. X-linked recessive: fathers cannot give it to sons and all daughters carry it.

5. X-linked dominant: mothers may give it to sons or daughters (50/50).

6. X-linked dominant: fathers cannot give it to sons and give it to all daughters.

7. Do not forget the occasional mitochondrial inheritance which comes only from mothers.

6.7 A 19-year-old girl asks to see you. Her brother has cystic fibrosis.

What is the approximate risk of her child having it?

6.8 You are asked to see a four-month-old girl who has lines of warts on her limbs. She was noted to have some vesicles in the first few days of life.

(a) What is the diagnosis?

(b) What is the mode of inheritance?

6.9 You are asked to see a 13-year-old girl because of her short stature. She has not entered puberty. Her LH/FSH are greatly raised.

(a) What is the diagnosis?

(b) How would you confirm this?

6.10

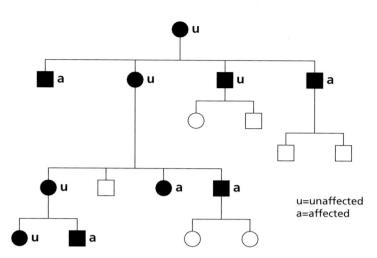

u=unaffected
a=affected

If this is not X-linked, what is the mode of inheritance?

6.11 You are reviewing a one-year-old child known to be hypertensive (127/65). He has the following investigation results:

Extra part of chromosome 15 on 19

Peripheral pulmonary branch stenosis

Horseshoe kidney – bilateral patchy uptake left 55% and right 45%.

(a) Why is he hypertensive?

(b) Name a possible treatment.

6.7 $\frac{2}{3} \times \frac{1}{4} \times \frac{1}{22} = \frac{1}{132}$

$\frac{2}{3}$ = Her chance of being a carrier.

$\frac{1}{4}$ = Chance of offspring having cystic fibrosis if both parents have it.

$\frac{1}{22}$ = Carrier rate (between $\frac{1}{20} - \frac{1}{25}$).

6.8 (a) Incontinentia pigmenti.

(b) X-linked dominant.

Comment: May also be presented as male deaths.

6.9 (a) Turner syndrome.

(b) Chromosomes looking for 45X0.

6.10 Mitochondrial.

Comment: Inheritance is only passed down the female line but to either sex.

6.11 (a) Scarring of the kidney = inappropriate angiotensin secretion.

(b) ACE inhibitor.

Comment: You are not being asked to show your knowledge of the chromosomal diagnosis.

Statistics

QUESTIONS (1)

7.1 A trial of a new test gives the following results:

	Has disease	Does not have disease
Positive	90	10
Negative	10	90

(a) What is the sensitivity?

(b) What is the specificity?

7.2 On auditing urine results you find the following:

	Pure growth organism	Multiple growth
> 50 WBC	95	15
< 50 WBC	10	200

(a) What is the positive predictive value?

(b) What is the negative predictive value?

7.1 (a) 90%

(b) 90%

7.2 (a) 95/110

(b) 200/210

Helpful hints

2 X 2 CHARTS

Sensitivity = the proportion of people with the condition that the test picks up.

Specificity = the proportion of people without the condition that have a negative test.

Positive predictive value = the chance that someone has the condition if the test is positive.

Negative predictive value = the chance that someone does not have the condition if the test is negative.

For example

Sensitivity	=	$\dfrac{a}{a+c}$
Specificity	=	$\dfrac{d}{d+b}$
Positive predictive value	=	$\dfrac{a}{a+b}$
Negative predictive value	=	$\dfrac{d}{d+c}$

	Have condition	*Do not have condition*
Positive test	a	b
Negative test	c	d

Comment: Make sure the chart is correctly orientated.

7.3 A test has a positive predictive value of 90 and a negative predictive value of 95. Draw an appropriate 2×2 table.

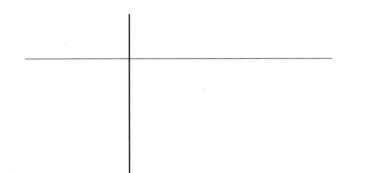

7.4 List five of the criteria for a screening programme.

7.3

	Have condition	Do not have condition
Positive	90	10
Negative	5	95

7.4 (a) The condition is a serious one.

(b) An acceptable test can pick up the condition before it is clinically detectable.

(c) The disease course can be altered by early detection.

(d) The test is highly sensitive and specific.

(e) The programme is cost effective.

Electrolytes

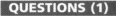

8

8.1 The following blood results were obtained from an 18-month-old failing to thrive.

Sodium   127 mmol/L

Potassium   2.6 mmol/L

Chloride   80 mmol/L

(a) What is the most likely diagnosis?

(b) What is the pathophysiology?

8.2 The following results occurred in a three-day-old 26-week gestation neonate while on a radiant warmer.

Sodium   147 mmol/L

Potassium   4.3 mmol/L

Urea   6.0 mmol/L

Creatinine 97 µmol/L

(a) What is the diagnosis?

_____

(b) Give two management strategies.

_____

_____

8.3 The following blood results were obtained on an ill six-year-old.

Sodium   135 mmol/L

Potassium   4.6 mmol/L

Urea   10.0 mmol/L

Osmolality 310 mOsm/kg

(a) What blood result is missing?

_____

(b) Approximately what should the result be?

_____

8.4 A 10-year-old diabetic is admitted semi-conscious. Urgent blood results are as follows:

Blood glucose	40$^+$ mmol/L
Osmolality	350 mOsm/kg
pH	7.26

What is the diagnosis?

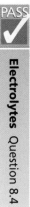

8.1 (a) Bartter syndrome.

(b) Vascular unresponsiveness to angiotensin; renal loss of chloride.

Comment: You need to always try to make the data fit the answer. In this case there is a low chloride; it may also give the pH. In Bartter the pH shows an alkalosis; Pseudo-Bartter may produce similar results but not enough information.

8.2 (a) Dehydration.

(b) Place in a humidified incubator and increase the fluids.

Comment: Always put answers in order of importance as they may include things like 're-check electrolytes later, cover with bubble sheet', and so on.

8.3 (a) Blood glucose.

(b) 20 mmol/L.

Comment: Whenever osmolality is mentioned, work out approximately what it should be, for example 2 × [Na + K] + urea + glucose – often one is missing in the question.

8.4 Non-ketotic hyperosmolar coma.

Comment: The high glucose would be appropriate for diabetic ketoacidosis (DKA) but you would expect a low pH if the patient was semi-conscious. ✔

Helpful hints

ELECTROLYTE AND DEXTROSE SOLUTIONS

1. Dextrose as mg/kg/h   (*should be / min !*)

$$= \frac{10 \times \% \text{ dextrose} \times \text{mL/h}}{\text{wt} \times 60}$$

For example, 1 kg neonate on 7.5% dextrose at 120 ml/kg/day

$$= \frac{10 \times 7.5 \times {}^{120}\!/_{24}}{60}$$

$$\text{mg/kg/h} = \frac{10 \times 7.5 \times 5}{60} = \frac{37.5}{6} = 6.25$$

Normal is 5 mg/kg/h. Only need to investigate if low BM and >12 mg/kg/h.

2. Sodium: formula to work out deficit

0.6 × deficit × wt in mmol/L

Be careful as dextrose is usually expressed in mg whereas everything else is in mmol.

3. 0.18% = 30 mmol/L

0.9% = 150 mmol/L

Note that 30% is usually easier to remember per millilitre = 5 mmol/ml

Examples

(a) 12 kg child with sodium 115 mmol/L

Normal 135 mmol/L $\Rightarrow$ deficit = $(135 - 115) \times 0.6 \times 12 = 144$ mmol

(b) Neonate on 1 ml/h of 0.45% saline

150 ml/kg/day of dextrose 10% + 0.18% saline

Is this neonate getting enough sodium?

(They usually need 4 mmol/kg/day)

Assume 1 kg

$$\Rightarrow \frac{(24 \times 75)}{1000} + \frac{(150 \times 30)}{1000} = 6.3 \text{ mmol/kg/day}$$

4. Potassium: 10 mmol/500 ml = 0.15% KCL

8.5 A child has a sodium of 118 mmol/L. The child weighs 20 kg and you want to increase his sodium to 135 mmol/L.

What is the deficit?

8.6 A seven-day-old neonate who is known to have septicaemia has the following results from his arterial line:

      Sodium   135 mmol/L

      Potassium   8.4 mmol/L

      Urea   12.4 mmol/L

      Creatinine   165 µmol/L

(a) What is the most likely cause of his high potassium?

(b) List three treatment options to bring it down.

8.7 A four-day-old 28-week gestation neonate had a blood sugar reading of 1.6 mmol/L and this was only stabilized on 150 mL/kg/day of 10% dextrose.

(a) Does this warrant further investigation?

_____

(b) Justify your answer.

_____

_____

8.8 You are asked to review a 29-week-gestation neonate who is one day old with poor urine output. The following results are available:

Hb	14.3 g/dL
WBC	3.5×10^9/L
Platelets	139×10^9/L
Sodium	127 mmol/L
Potassium	3.3 mmol/L

(a) What is the most likely diagnosis and cause?

_____

(b) What fluid management is appropriate?

_____

8.9 A 1-kg baby is receiving the following i.v. fluids:

UAC 0.45% NaCl 1 mL/h

Peripheral line 200 mL/kg/day of dextrose 10%. + 0.18% NaCl

How many mmol/kg of sodium is this baby on?

8.5 $(135 - 118) \times 0.6 \times 20 = 204$ mmol

Comment: See hints.

8.6   (a) Acute pre-renal failure.

(b) Fluid bolus.

  i.v. B dextrose and insulin

  Intravenous salbutamol.

Comment: Try to expand renal failure to fit with the history given.

8.7   (a) No.

(b)

$$\frac{\cancel{10} \times \cancel{10}^{5} \times \dfrac{\cancel{150}^{\,\cancel{6}\,2}}{\cancel{24}}}{\cancel{60}_{\,\cancel{3}\ 1}} = 10 \text{ mg/kg/h}$$

Do not investigate until >12 mg/kg/h.

Comment: Write down the calculation so that you may get some marks, even if it is slightly wrong.

8.8   (a) Inappropriate ADH secondary to sepsis.

(b) Fluid restriction.

Comment: Poor urine output is often because neonates are dehydrated, but here the sodium is low.

8.9 (a) Umbilical artery catheter (UAC) 24 ml/day

0.45% NaCl = 75 mmol/L

$$\frac{\overset{3}{\cancel{24}}}{\underset{\underset{5}{40}}{\cancel{1000}}} \times \overset{3}{\cancel{75}} = \frac{9}{5} \text{ mmol}$$

(b) Peripheral line 150 ml/day

0.18% = 30 mmol/L

$$\frac{\cancel{200}}{\cancel{1000}} \times 3\cancel{0} = 6 \text{ mmol}$$

Total = 7.8 mmol

Emergency medicine

9

9.1 You are crash called to a two-year-old in the Accident and Emergency department who is unresponsive to initial attempts to resuscitate.

(a) How much would you expect him to weigh?

(b) What is an appropriate dose of adrenaline if administrated via the endotracheal tube?

9.2 A five-year-old child in intensive care is intubated with intravenous access, but has a cardiac arrest.

(a) What are the first two things to do?

(b) What is the intravenous dose of adrenaline?

9.3 A three-year-old patient has a prolonged febrile convulsion.

(a) What is the rectal dose of diazepam?

(b) What is the loading dose of phenytoin?

9.4 You are urgently called to A&E to see a six-week-old baby who is centrally cyanosed, but not in distress. The casualty officer has started facial oxygen and the saturations are 76%.

(a) What is the most likely diagnosis?

(b) What is your first action?

9.5 The following blood gas was obtained from a sick eight-year-old:

pH   7.15

Anion gap   40 mmol/L

K^+ 5.7 mmol/L

What is the likely diagnosis?

9.6 A pre-term neonate is being ventilated for respiratory distress syndrome on the following setting:

Rate   60 BPM

Inspiration   0.3 sec

Pressure   24/4

O_2 40%

He is active and over the course of 15 min his oxygen requirement goes up.

His gas is:

pH   7.1

PCO_2 90 mm/Hg

PO_2 45 mm/Hg

(a) Give three possible explanations for this change.

(b) Give management instructions in appropriate order.

9.7 A neonate who has been ventilated for two days has a base deficit of 16. He has had a bolus of saline and you want to give him bicarbonate. He is 1.5 kg.

How much is a half correction of his acidosis?

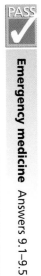

9.1 (a) (Age + 4) × 2 = 12 kg

✓(b) 0.1 ml/kg of 1 in 1000 = 1.2 mL

Comment: All emergency medicine follows national recognized guidelines – learn them.

9.2 (a) Check airway and breathing.

(b) First dose — 0.1 mL/kg of 1 in 10000 = 1.8 mL

Subsequent dose 1.8 mL of 1 in 1000

Comment: In part (b) there are two lines so there should be two answers. If the examiners provide two lines for an answer, which they would in (b), make sure you give two answers.

9.3 (a) 14 × 0.4 mg = 5.6 mg

(b) 14 × 18 mg = 252 mg but only if not already on phenytoin.

Comment: Writing the extra guide in (b) shows a greater understanding.

9.4 (a) Congenital heart disease.

(b) Stop the oxygen.

Comment: The child is blue but happy.

9.5 Diabetic ketoacidosis.

Comment: Acidosis with increased anion gap.

9.6 (a) Blocked/dislodged tube

Pneumothorax

Worsening disease

(b) (i) Listen to air entry.

(ii) Cold light chest to exclude pneumothorax.

(iii) Re-intubate as needed and then increase ventilation setting.

Comment: Think also sepsis and interventricular haemorrhage. If there is co-ordination with the ventilator you may need to increase sedation.

9.7 $0.5 \times 1.5 \times 16 = 8 \times 1.5 = 12$ mL of 8.4% bicarbonate.

Comment: Do not try and be clever, suggesting THAM. Make sure the bicarbonate concentration is there. You can mention that you would dilute to 4.2% with water.

Helpful hints

BLOOD GASES

✱ 1. Always convert the gas into the units you are used to, using the factor 7.5.

For example mm Hg = $\underline{7.5 \times kPa}$

2. Make sure the diagnosis fits the age of the patient.

For example:

✓Alkalosis in a six-week-old? Think pyloric stenosis.

✓Alkalosis in a teenager? Think aspirin.

3. Decide whether the gas demonstrates a respiratory or a metabolic problem.

If it is metabolic with normal anion gap it is either RTA or pyloric stenosis.

4. Neonatal causes

Respiratory acidosis	Metabolic acidosis
• RDS	• Sepsis
• Pneumothorax	• Dehydrated
• Blocked tube	• Renal
• Pneumonia	• Metabolic
	• Cardiac
	• IVH

5. **NB** Raised CO_2 with cyanosis is rarely cardiac.

9.8 A three-day-old with RDS is improving when you are asked to review the following arterial gas.

pH	7.29
PCO_2	70 mmHg
PO_2	80 mmHg
BE	–6 mmol/L

What would you like to do?

9.9 A six-hour-old 27-weeker is ventilated with a rate of 50 BPM when you are asked to review the following gas:

pH	7.25
PCO_2	58 mmHg
PO_2	76 mmHg

The baby is in 60% oxygen and has intermittent unco-ordinated respirations

List three treatment options.

9.10 You are crash called to the emergency room where a four-year-old, who has fallen through the ice on a frozen pond, is in ventricular fibrillation.

(a) Give the appropriate defibrillation settings for three shocks.

(b) List three measures to warm him.

9.8   Repeat gas.

Comment: Raised CO_2 would need a positive base excess to have a pH of 7.29, so it must be wrong.

9.9   Increase the rate.

Increase the sedation.

Paralyse.

Comment: Try to decide the order you would use in practice.

9.10 (a) $2 \times wt = 32 \, j$

   $2 \times wt = 32 \, j$

   $4 \times wt = 64 \, j$

(b) Remove wet clothing

   Warm blankets

   Warm i.v. fluids

   Peritoneal warming (or bladder/stomach)

   Cardiac bypass

NB Do not use a space blanket – it *keeps* warm but does not warm.

Haematology

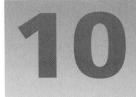

10.1 Further investigation of a three-year-old with suspected
platelet disease has the following results:

On film platelets appear normal

Normal aggregation to ADP and collagen

But abnormal aggregation to ristocetin

What is the likely diagnosis?

10.2 A four-month-old is thought to be pale when seen by a GP.

A full blood count is taken:

Hb   4.6 g/dL

WCC $11.2 \times 10^9/L$

Platelets $225 \times 10^9/L$

Reticulocytes 0.5%

(a) Suggest a possible diagnosis.

_____

(b) How would you confirm it?

_____

10.3 A four-year-old being investigated for anaemia had the following electrophoresis results:

HbA   85%

HbA_2 5%

HbF   3%

What is the reason for his anaemia?

_____

10.4 A six-year-old boy suffering from recurrent infections with associated eczema has his FBC checked:

     Hb   12.1 g/dL

     WCC 10.6×10^9/L

     Platelets 45×10^9/L

(a) What is the likely diagnosis?

(b) What are the immunoglobulin levels (IgA, IgE, IgM)?

10.5 An Asian child is suspected of having α-thalassaemia. FBC shows he has a mean cell haemoglobin (MCH) of 30 pg.

Does he need further investigation?

✓ **10.6** You are asked to see a two-year-old girl who complains of back pain and has a history of frequent illness. Her mother feels she has been pale for about six months. FBC:

Hb	5.7 g/dL
WCC	7.3×10^9/L
Platelets	352×10^9/L
MCV	78 fL
Blood film	Normal

(a) What is your primary concern?

_____

(b) List two further investigations you would make.

_____

_____

10.7 ✓ You are asked to see a child with a rash. Your clinical diagnosis is urticarial but because of marked bruising you ask for a FBC:

Hb	9.3 g/dL
WCC	10.4×10^9/L
Platelets	232×10^9/L
MCH	22.4 pg
MCV	69.6 fL
Zinc protoporphyrin	63 μmol ZPP/mol heme
HbA$_2$	3.9 (2.1–3.4%)
√HbF	2.6 (< 0.8%)

(a) What is the diagnosis?

_____

(b) Can this present as neonatal jaundice?

_____

10.8 You review a three-year-old with lower back pain who has poor appetite and drinks 4–5 pints of milk a day. She is thriving. The results of a FBC:

Hb   10.1 g/L

WCC 4.4×10^9/L

Platelets 227×10^9/L

MCV   68.5 fL

(a) What is the likely diagnosis?

(b) What confirmatory blood test is there?

10.9 You are reviewing a four-year-old with bruises. There is a history of a pyrexial illness with red cheeks.

Hb   12.6 g/dL

WCC 2.5×10^9/L

Platelets 10×10^9/L

(a) What illness has she had?

(b) What is the causative agent?

10.10 You are asked to see a 10-year-old child in Outpatients whose father is Chinese. He has presented with non-specific abdominal pain.

Hb	11.8 g/dL
MCV	70.6 fL
MCH	22.1 pg
HbA$_2$	2.8 (normal 2.1–3.4%)
HbF	0.5 (< 0.8%)
Zinc protoporphyrin	43 (normal 0–80) μmol ZPP/mol heme
Film	Microcytosis, hypochromia

(a) What is the likely diagnosis?

(b) Is it causing her abdominal pain?

(c) What neonatal problems may it cause?

10.11 You are asked to see a jaundiced baby on day 1.

Bilirubin   110 µmol/L

Baby's blood group   O Rh positive

Mother's blood group   O Rh negative

Mother tells you that she has had a splenectomy.

(a) Give two possible diagnoses.

(b) Give two differentiating tests.

10.12 You are reviewing a thriving two-year-old in clinic with a 2 cm spleen and a family history of spherocytosis. FBC results:

Hb	9.0 g/dL
WCC	10.4×10^9/L
MCV	29 fL
Platelets	422×10^9/L
Zinc protoporphyrin	87 (0–80) µmol ZPP/mol heme
Reticulocytes	10.2%

(a) Name one medication this child should be given.

(b) If this child needs a splenectomy give two management requirements.

✓ **10.13** A two-year-old has been in for six days with a pyrexia, cough and a fine macular rash which seems to appear with the evening rise in temperature. Palpable spleen 2 cm.

Hb	8.1 g/dL
WCC	17.4×10^9/L
MCV	70.6 fL
Platelets	606×10^9/L
ESR	120 mm/h

(a) What is the most likely diagnosis?

(b) What would be your initial treatment?

10.14 A 2½ year old with Still's disease is not well controlled so is admitted for a bone marrow biopsy.

(a) Why has he had a bone marrow biopsy?

(b) How would you monitor the Still's disease?

10.1 (a) Von Willebrand.

Comment: Normal size platelets; if large then consider Bernard Soulier.

10.2 (a) Blackfan–Diamond syndrome.

(b) Bone marrow biopsy.

Comment: Best fit to age, may also mention hypoplasia of the thumb.

10.3 β-thalassaemia trait.

Comment: The presence of HbF tells you it is β and the presence of HbA tells you it is trait.

10.4 (a) Wiskott–Aldrich syndrome.

(b) IgA↑ IgE↑ IgM↓

Comment: There is a group of syndromes with altered immunoglobulin levels but there is no logic to them so they have to be learnt.

10.5 No.

Comment: You only need to investigate if it is less than 27 pg.

10.6 (a) Malignancy.

(b) MRI scan of spine

Bone marrow biopsy.

Comment: It is very unusual for a child to complain of back pain. It may also be infection but in view of the low haemoglobin, the prime concern is malignancy.

10.7 (a) β-thalassaemia.

(b) No.

Comment: Increased HbA_2 + HbF β chains are not present at birth so do not cause neonatal problems.

10.8 (a) Iron deficiency anaemia.

(b) Zinc protoporphyrin levels or ferretin levels.

Comment: Milk allows a baby to thrive but is a very poor source of iron.

10.9 (a) Fifth disease of childhood (slapped cheek syndrome or erythema infectiosum).

(b) Parvovirus B19.

10.10 (a) α-thalassaemia trait.

(b) No.

(c) Neonatal hydrops

Interuterine death.

Comment: Low normal haemoglobin with a very low mean cell haemoglobin is usually either thalassaemia or iron deficiency.

10.11 (a) Rhesus incompatibility

Spherocytosis

(b) Direct Coombs test

Blood film

Red cell fragility test

Comment: In (a) the order is, probably, not relevant as both are likely.

In (b) two tests are needed that differentiate between your diagnosis in (a).

10.12 (a) Folic acid. (Fewer marks for iron.)

(b) Pneumococcal/meningococcal/haemophilus B vaccination – encapsulated organisms.

Prophylactic penicillin.

Comment: The reticulocyte count is much higher than the zinc protoporphyrin level. In (b), do not put down two vaccinations.

10.13 (a) Systemic juvenile arthritis.

(b) NSAIDs.

Comment: Evening rise of temperature is the clue here.

10.14 (a) To exclude leukaemia before starting oral steroids.

(b) ESR

Platelets

Clinically.

Comment: All children who are going on to steroids need a biopsy – that includes those with idiopathic thrombocytopenia purpura (ITP).

Gastro-enterology

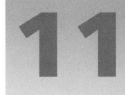

QUESTIONS (1)

11.1 You are reviewing a two-year-old with a family history of coeliac disease, who is not thriving.

Total protein	50 g/L
IgA	< 0.2 g/L
Anti-endomysial antibodies	Not detected

Please comment.

11.2 A four-week-old is referred because of mild jaundice. She is breast-fed and feeding well.

Bilirubin total	110 µmol/L
Indirect	20 µmol/L

What is the most likely diagnosis?

11.3 You are requested to do the following investigation on a three-year-old who is chesty.

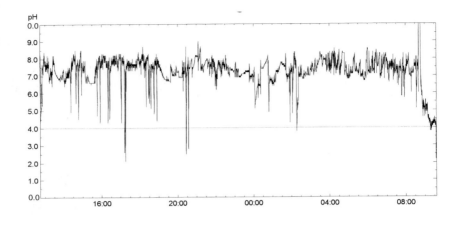

(a) What is the investigation?

_____

(b) Have you found the reason for his chestiness?

_____

11.4 The tracing below was taken from a child who has been having frequent abscences. These were thought to have been caused by reflux.

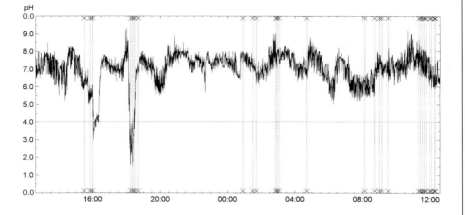

(a) Are there any indications of reflux?

(b) Is reflux the cause of these episodes?

11.5 The child below has cerebral palsy. He is to have a percutaneous endoscopic gastrostomy (PEG).

(a) Is he having the right operation?

(b) Justify your answer.

11.6 You are reviewing a six-month-old baby with constipation. There is some improvement with lactulose and senna. Reviewing his notes he was initially breast-fed and first opened his bowels on day 6.

What would you do next?

11.7 A four-year-old with an acute abdomen has the following findings:

Abdomen: Tender on the right, bowel sounds present

FBC:

Hb	15 g/dL
WCC	20×10^9/L (90% neutrophils)
Platelets	400×10^9/L
Amylase	650 IU/L
Ultrasound	Free fluid – 2.5 cm mass behind the bladder

(a) What is the diagnosis?

_____

(b) Give two possible aetiologies.

_____

_____

(c) Give one complication.

_____

11.1 Anti-endomysial is IgA, so as the IgA levels are very low it is not a useful test. The child needs a jejunal biopsy.

11.2 Biliary atresia.

Comment: Do not be fooled when you are given results that you are not used to, for example indirect bilirubin.

11.3 (a) 24 h oesophageal pH.

(b) No.

11.4 (a) Minimal evidence, as only two episodes are below pH 4.0.

(b) No: the lines are episodes of absence and they are not related to reflux.

11.5 (a) No

(b) The 24 h pH recording has demonstrated numerous episodes of reflux. It is not possible to perform an anti-reflux procedure such as Nissan's with an endoscope. Reflux should normally be less than 10% of the total times.

11.6 Take a rectal biopsy to rule out Hirschsprung's.

11.7 (a) Pancreatitis.

(b) Mumps, cystic fibrosis, trauma.

(c) Pseudocyst.

Syndromes

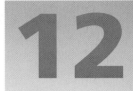

QUESTIONS (1)

√ **12.1** A three-week-old baby presents with vomiting and diarrhoea.

An observant SHO notices lens clouding.

(a) What is the most likely diagnosis?

_____

(b) Name a confirmatory test.

_____

 12.2 A three-year-old child with learning difficulties is referred to you by the ophthalmologist.

(a) What is the most likely diagnosis?

_____

(b) Name a confirmatory test on the urine.

_____

12.3 A 10-year-old is referred to you for intermittent mild jaundice. His urine and stools are normal.

(a) What is the most likely diagnosis?

(b) What is the mode of inheritance?

12.4 A seven-year-old girl is referred with tiredness and symmetrical proximal muscle weakness. There is some tenderness.

(a) Give two other features you would look for.

(b) What is the mainstay of treatment?

12.5 You are asked to see a three-year-old boy who has pubic hair and an enlarged penis. His electrolytes, however, are normal.

What is the most likely diagnosis?

12.1   (a) Galactosaemia

(b) Galactose-1-phosphate uridyl transferase (Gal-i-put) blood test.

Comment: Give the full test names.

12.2   (a) Homocystinuria.

(b) Homocystine levels.

Comment: Other syndromes have eye changes, but the diagnosis needs to be made on a urine sample.

12.3   (a) Gilbert syndrome.

(b) Autosomal recessive.

12.4   (a) Facial purple helitropic rash; oedema in hands or feet; subcutaneous nodules.

(b) Steroids.

Comment: The child has dermatomyositis.

12.5   Non-salt-losing congenital adrenal hyperplasia.

Comment: Use all the information in the question. Adrenal pubertal growth does not affect the testes or ovaries as they are controlled by LH/FSH.

PASS ✓

Helpful hints

SYNDROMES

1. The syndromes that you remember are the ones that you have seen.

2. To facilitate this there are two options:

   (a) Go to your local special schools even before the clinical part of this examination;

   (b) After answering any question on syndromes take notes then look in the syndrome book.

3. 2(a) is the best option as most syndromes that you will be asked about rarely come in as patients.

4. These questions are quite common in the slide section and Hint no. 2 helps because features run true. It is not wasted time.

12.6 A seven-year-old with acne is referred to you. You notice that she is obese.

(a) What is the most likely diagnosis?

(b) Give two other clinical features.

12.7 A 13-year-old girl is referred to you through the school nurse because she looks tired although she says she doesn't feel it.

(a) What is a possible diagnosis?

(b) Give two treatment options.

✓ **12.8** You are referred an eight-year-old boy who has hypermobile joints. There is a history of numerous abscesses.

(a) What is the most likely diagnosis?

(b) Name one possible treatment.

12.9 You are reviewing a child with obesity in follow up clinic. Reading his notes you see that a plastic surgeon has seen him for polydactyly. He has also been diagnosed as having visual problems.

(a) What is the underlying diagnosis?

(b) Explain his visual problems.

12.10 You are asked to see an 18-month-old who was developing normally until seven months of age. Autism has been suggested but the child's condition is getting worse. There are hyperventilation episodes and head growth has slowed.

(a) What is the diagnosis?

_____

(b) What sex is the child?

_____

12.6 (a) Cushing syndrome.

(b) Stretch marks

Hirsutism

Comment: Increased BP would not be a clinical feature.

12.7 (a) Myasthenia gravis

(b) Neostigmine

Thymectomy

Comment: Thymectomy fits with female sex.

12.8 (a) Job syndrome.

(b) Cimetidine.

Comment: It is also known as hyper-IgE syndrome.

12.9 (a) Laurence–Moon–Biedl.

(b) Retinitis pigmentosa.

12.10 (a) Rett syndrome.

(b) Female.

Comment: When asked what sex a child is do not assume the child is male!

Miscellaneous

13

13.1 A 12-year-old boy presents to you with a painful left leg. There is some restriction of movement.

(a) What is the most likely diagnosis?

(b) What is the investigation of choice?

13.2 A three-year-old presents with a limp and pain that wakes her at night. The hip X-ray is normal and so is the FBC and ESR.

What is the next investigation?

13.3

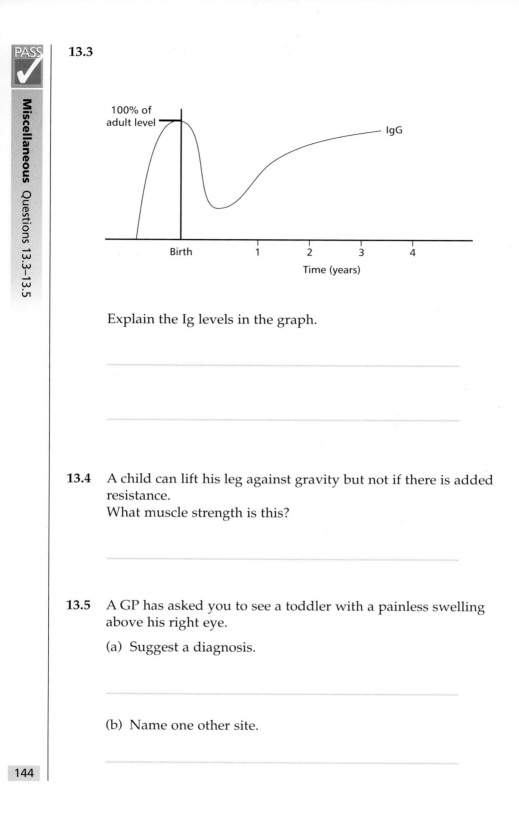

Explain the Ig levels in the graph.

_____

_____

13.4 A child can lift his leg against gravity but not if there is added resistance.
What muscle strength is this?

_____

13.5 A GP has asked you to see a toddler with a painless swelling above his right eye.

(a) Suggest a diagnosis.

_____

(b) Name one other site.

_____

13.6 A baby is born with a swelling of the left side of the scrotum. Over the next 24 h it goes blue/black.

(a) What is the diagnosis?

(b) What is the prognosis?

(c) Does the child need an operation?

13.7 Two children have their visual fields tested.

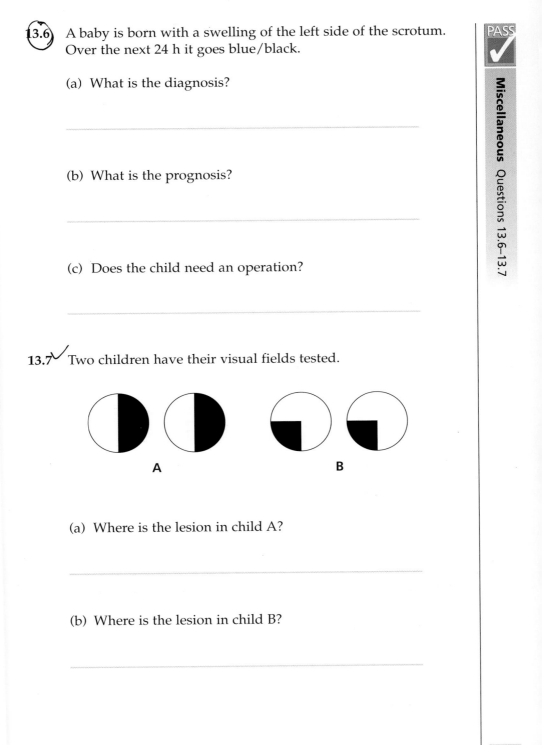

A   B

(a) Where is the lesion in child A?

(b) Where is the lesion in child B?

13.8 You are asked to review the following cell count from a lumbar puncture undertaken on a 12-year-old boy.

RBC	$214\,000 \times 10^6/L$
WBC	$396 \times 10^6/L$

Is it significant?

13.9 A nine-year-old girl initially presents with some facial weakness. The following lumbar puncture result is available:

WCC	$< 5 \times 10^6/L$
Protein	2.2 g/L
Glucose	3.6 mmol/L

(a) What is the diagnosis?

(b) What monitoring is most important?

13.10 A 15-month-old is admitted; she is refusing to walk and has prominence of the spine in the thoraco-lumbar area. She is apyrexial and not distressed.

FBC:

Hb	11.4 g/dL
WCC	11.5×10^9/L
Platelets	415×10^9/L
CRP	12 mg/L

Plain X-ray of spine erosion   L1–L2

What are the main differential diagnoses?

13.1 (a) Slipped femoral epiphysis on the left.

(b) Lateral hip X-ray.

Comment: Fit the diagnosis with the patient's age. He would need to be younger for Perthes' (4–8 years of age).

13.2 X-ray the rest of the leg.

Comment: Pathology may have been missed, for example Ewing's sarcoma.

13.3 The first rise is transplacental IgG which dips before the baby starts producing its own.

13.4 3/5

0 – No movement

1 – Slight movement

2 – Movement, but not against gravity

3 – Movement against gravity

4 – Near normal

5 – Normal

13.5 (a) Dermoid.

(b) Many places commonly anterior to the ear or the middle of the neck.

13.6 (a) Congenital torsion.

(b) The swelling will settle leaving a palpable remnant only.

(c) No.

Comment: Congenital torsion is usually on the left and, unlike torsion in the older age group, the other testis does not need fixing.

13.7 (a) Left optic tract.

(b) Right parietal lobe.

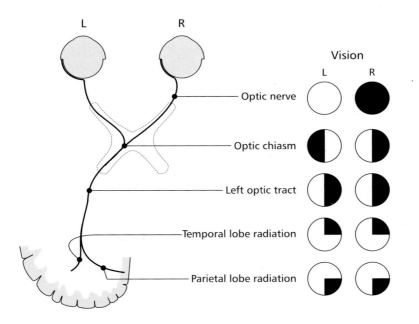

Comment: Whenever answering a question on visual pathways, draw the pathway.

13.8 (a) No.

Comment: One WBC for 500 RBC = $\dfrac{214000}{500}$ = 428

13.9 (a) Guillain–Barré syndrome.

(b) Respiratory function using a spirometer.

Comment: Question (b) removes any uncertainty to question (a).

13.10 Discitis

Tumour

Comment: In view of non-raised CRP it is difficult to put the answers in order.

Exam 1

14

14.1 A cardiologist is reviewing a two-year-old with a systolic murmur. He is noted to have some soft dysmorphic features.

ECG – normal

Echo – mild supravalvular aortic stenosis

(a) What is the likely diagnosis?

(b) Give one other cardiac lesion.

(c) What blood test may be abnormal in the neonatal period?

(d) What is the confirmatory test?

14.2 A 15-year-old is admitted with meningitis. While in hospital he has audiometry tests.

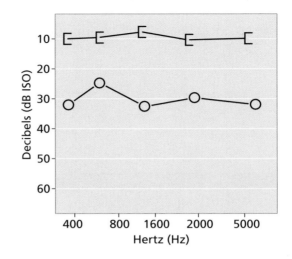

(a) Does he need an operation?

_____

(b) Justify your answer.

_____

✓**14.3** A five-year-old with known renal tubular acidosis has the following test result.

Bicarbonate loading – urine more alkaline

Which type of RTA does he have?

_____

✓
14.4 A boy presents to you in Outpatients with a one-week history of a cough; he is also pyrexial. He has a history of frequent skin abscesses and intermittent diarrhoea.

(a) What would you expect his immunoglobulins to be (IgA, IgM, IgG)?

(b) What is the inheritance?

(c) Name one confirmatory test.

(d) What treatment may be required?

Exam 1 Question 14.4

PASS

14.5 A newly diagnosed diabetic has high pre-breakfast blood sugars, but is also noted to be sweaty in the night.

(a) What is the diagnosis?

(b) What is the treatment plan?

14.6 A baby on the neonatal unit with prolonged jaundice is found to have a TSH of 150 mU/L.

Name two associated syndromes.

14.7 This is the family tree of a girl under your care. Her parents both have the same condition.

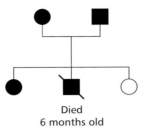

Died
6 months old

(a) What is the condition?

_____

(b) What caused her brother's death?

_____

14.8 A six-year-old presents to the department with a pyrexia and neck stiffness.

LP result

RBC   21 × 10⁶/L

WBC   264 × 10⁶/L

Gram positive diplococcus

(a) What is the likely organism?

_____

(b) Suggest an antibiotic.

_____

(c) What would you expect the glucose to be?

_____

_____

(14.9) A two-year-old girl is admitted with a two-month history of polyuria and polydipsia. She also vomits intermittently and has gained weight.

On admission   Glycosuria ✓

Blood sugar   11.2 mmol/L

Blood gas   Normal

Overnight   BMs 4–7 mmol/L

Next morning   Blood sugar 4.6 mmol/L

(a) What is the most likely diagnosis?

_____

(b) What is the management?

_____

14.10 A 6½-year-old is referred to you because of her short stature. The following results are available.

FBC	Normal
U&Es	Normal
GH	110 mU/L
TSH	Normal

(a) What is the likely diagnosis?

_____

(b) What is the mode of inheritance?

_____

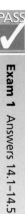

14.1 (a) Williams syndrome.

(b) Peripheral pulmonary artery stenosis or pulmonary valve stenosis.

(c) Hypercalcaemia.

(d) FISH deletion chromosome 7.

14.2 (a) No (not with the information given).

(b) The tests show mild right conductive hearing loss. The worry in meningitis is sensorineuronal loss.

14.3 Proximal renal tubular acidosis.

Comment: Acid or base loading will not change the pH in distal renal tubular acidosis.

14.4 (a) All raised.

(b) X-linked.

(c) Nitroblue tetrazolium dye reduction test.

(d) Antibiotics, white cell transfusion, bone marrow transplant.

Comment: He has chronic granulomatous disease.

14.5 (a) Somogyi affect.

(b) Decrease evening insulin.

Comment: Too much insulin causes nocturnal hypoglycaemia with compensatory growth hormone and cortisol surges. As the influence of exogenous insulin diminishes early morning hyperglycaemia occurs.

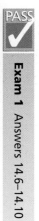

14.6 Down syndrome

Pendred syndrome.

14.7 (a) Achondroplasia.

(b) Constrictive thoracic dystrophy.

Comment: Caused by the do<u>ub</u>le dominant.

14.8 (a) Pneumococcus.

(b) Ceftriaxone, cefotaxime etc., or penicillin.

(c) Low/less than 40% of the blood glucose.

Comment: Part (c) has left a couple of lines, so you need to bring out the relationship with the blood glucose.

14.9 (a) Psychogenic polydipsia.

(b) Gradual decrease in fluids.

Comment: Does not fit with diabetes as blood gas is normal and settles with no treatment. Hugh glucose can be caused by glucose drinks.

14.10 (a) Laron dwarfism: end organ growth hormone insensitivity

(b) Autosomal recessive.

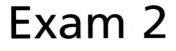

Exam 2

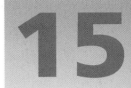

QUESTIONS

15.1 This is the spirometer reading of an eight-year-old girl.

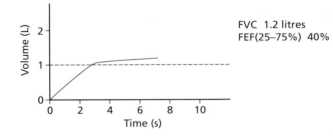

FVC 1.2 litres
FEF(25–75%) 40%

(a) What condition does she have?

_____

(b) What would you expect her FEV_1 to be?

_____

15.2 How old are these children? State their age by their ability to do the following.

(a) Make a tower of five bricks. _____

(b) Copy a flight of stairs out of building blocks. _____

(c) Draw

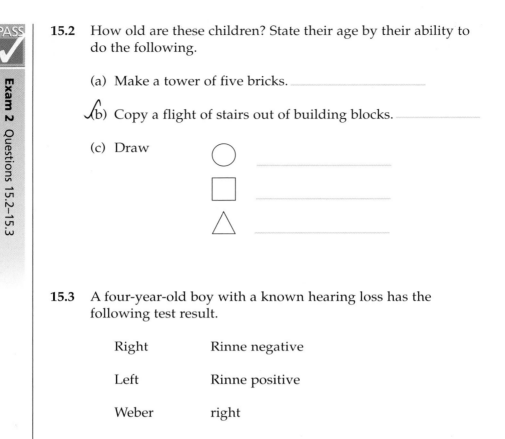

15.3 A four-year-old boy with a known hearing loss has the following test result.

Right	Rinne negative
Left	Rinne positive
Weber	right

(a) What hearing loss does he have?

_____

(b) What is his bone conduction on the affected side?

_____

15.4 Two unrelated families have had the same spontaneous mutation.

Family 1   Family 2

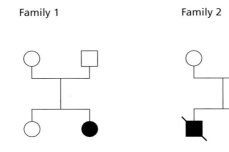

(a) What is the condition?

_____

(b) What is the mode of inheritance?

_____

15.5 A 15-year-old diabetic with well-controlled diabetes starts drinking excessively and passing a lot of urine.

What is the underlying diagnosis?

_____

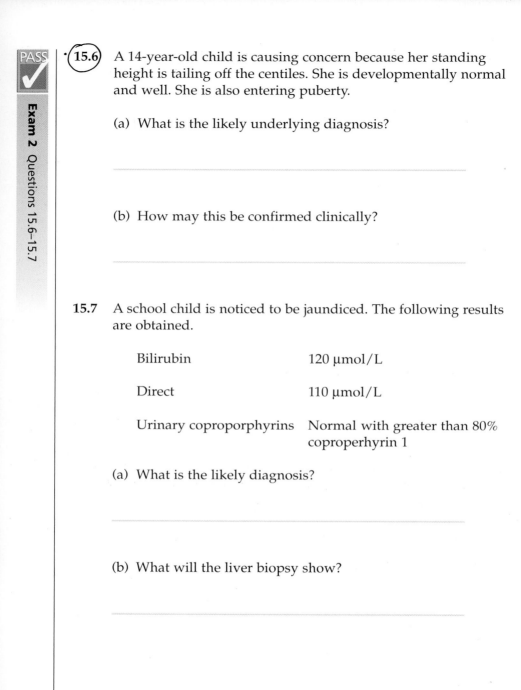

15.6 A 14-year-old child is causing concern because her standing height is tailing off the centiles. She is developmentally normal and well. She is also entering puberty.

(a) What is the likely underlying diagnosis?

(b) How may this be confirmed clinically?

15.7 A school child is noticed to be jaundiced. The following results are obtained.

Bilirubin	120 µmol/L
Direct	110 µmol/L
Urinary coproporphyrins	Normal with greater than 80% coproperhyrin 1

(a) What is the likely diagnosis?

(b) What will the liver biopsy show?

✓
15.8 A 3½-year-old is brought to you with obesity. He also has undescended testes. In the neonatal period he needed tube feeding.

(a) What is the most likely diagnosis?

(b) What are the two modes of inheritance?

(c) Which mode is more common?

15.9 A 2½-year-old is referred to your clinic because of irritability and sweatiness. There has been poor weight gain in the last six months.

(a) What is the diagnosis?

(b) Suggest a treatment.

(c) What is the natural history?

15.10 An eight-year-old boy is under your care and is having a glycogen stimulation test.

Time (sec)	GH (mU/L)	Cortisol (nmol/L)
0	6.4	93
30	5.4	270
60	2.6	187
90	1.1	120
120	2.8	125
180	7.2	184

(a) What does the test show?

(b) What is your management plan?

15.1 (a) Asthma.

(b) Markedly reduced.

15.2 (a) Two years.

(b) Four years.

(c) Three years, 5-and-a-half years, 4-and-a-half years.

Comment: Unfortunately this just has to be learned!

15.3 (a) Conduction hearing loss on the right.

(b) Normal.

Comment: Remember Rinne negative is always the abnormal ear.

15.4 (a) Incontinentia pigmenti.

(b) X-linked dominant.

15.5 DIDMOAD syndrome

Comment: Diabetes insipidus is the diagnosis but the above is the underlying diagnosis.

DI   = diabetic insipidus

DM = diabetes mellitus

OA = optic atrophy

D   = deafness

15.6 (a) Hypochondroplasia.

(b) Sitting height.

Comment: Shortening of limbs becomes more obvious at puberty. Sitting height nearer normal.

15.7 (a) Dubin–Johnson syndrome.

(b) Normal.

15.8 (a) Prader–Willi syndrome.

(b) Paternal deletion

Maternal disomy.

(c) Paternal deletion.

Comment: Paternal deletion/maternal disomy = Prader–Willi syndrome. Paternal disomy/maternal deletion = Angelman syndrome.

15.9 (a) Hyperthyroidism.

(b) Carbimazole propranolol.

(c) The child will grow out of it.

15.10 (a) GH and cortisol deficiency.

(b) GH supplementation: 1 im injection 6 days a week; Cortisol supplementation: ⅔ morning, ⅓ evening; increased with illness and early admission if vomiting.

Comment: (b) tells you the answer to (a) but you can also write too much in (b), so try to get a couple of points down for both GH and cortisol replacement.

Exam 3

QUESTIONS

16.1 An eight-year-old boy is admitted with a painful left ankle associated with a limp. There was also some pain in the left wrist. On examination he looks well and is apyrexial. There is no obvious swelling. The pain settled with ibuprofen. There was a history of a mild sore throat about three weeks ago.

Hb	12.4 g/dL
WCC	10.6×10^9/L
Platelets	474×10^9/L
ESR	56×10^9/L
Rh factor	< 20 mm/h

Anti-nuclear antibodies Negative

He is still well one year later.

Give the most likely diagnosis.

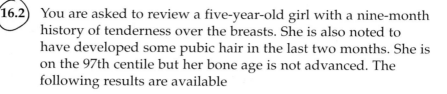

16.2 You are asked to review a five-year-old girl with a nine-month history of tenderness over the breasts. She is also noted to have developed some pubic hair in the last two months. She is on the 97th centile but her bone age is not advanced. The following results are available

TSH	2.2	mU/L
Oestradiol	400	pmol/L
Prolactin	131	(Normal 0–450 mU/L)

LHRH test		LH (U/L)	FSH (U/L)
time (min)	0	< 1	40
	30	22.0	19.2
	60	14.3	19.9

(a) What do the tests show?

(b) What other investigation is necessary and why?

16.3 A four-year-old child with a positive family history of spherocytosis undergoes an osmotic fragility test.

Mean cell fragility   fresh 4.6 g/l NaCl (4–4.45)

post-incubation 6.6 g/l NaCl (4.65–5.9)

Has the child got spherocytosis?

16.4 A two-year-old boy is admitted with a swollen face and abdominal distension of seven days' standing. He has been treated for a sore throat.

Hb	12.2 g/dL
WCC	$13.9 \times 10^9/L$
Platelets	$547 \times 10^9/L$
Urea	3.3 mmol/L
Sodium	138 mmol/L
BP	120/70 mmHg
Albumin	16 g/L
Urine protein	+++

(a) What is the likely diagnosis?

(b) What is the initial treatment?

(c) What is the long-term course?

√16.5 On holiday, a five-year-old presents with haematuria. There is no history of illness and he is well.

Urine

    RBC   Uncountable

    WBC $< 20\ 10^6/L$

    No organisms seen

Blood

    Hb   12.4 g/dL

    WCC $10.1 \times 10^9/L$

    Platelets $232 \times 10^9/L$

    Sodium   136 mmol/L

    Potassium   4.6 mmol/L

    Urea   3.2 mmol/L

    Albumin   44 g/L

(a) Give three possible diagnoses.

(b) Name three further observations/investigations.

_____

_____

_____

√16.6 You are reviewing a nine-year-old in clinic whom you have been treating with vasopressin for four years. You have just plotted his height and weight (see chart).

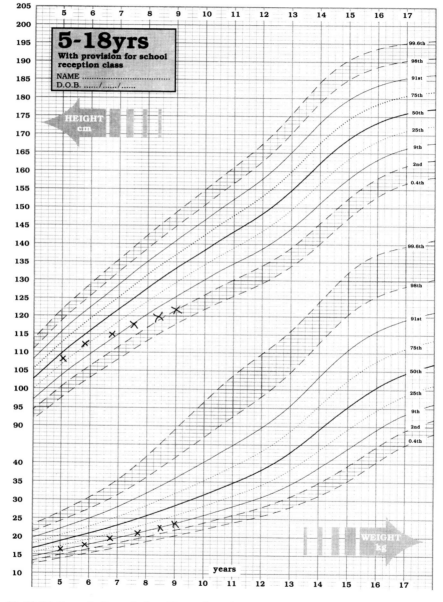

(© Child Growth Foundation. Reproduced with permission.)

(a) Give a likely diagnosis for the growth chart.

_____

(b) Give an underlying diagnosis.

_____

(c) Name two other tests you should do.

_____

_____

16.7 A 10-year-old boy is admitted to A&E unable to walk and complaining of pain in his thighs. He has previously been fit and well.

Hb	14.0 g/dL
WBC	3.1×10^9/L
Neutrophils	1.3×10^9/L
Platelets	128×10^9/L
Potassium	4.4 mmol/L
Urea	4.4 mmol/L
CPK	2987 IU/L

(a) What is the likely diagnosis?

(b) What is the prognosis?

16.8 The following results are from a sample of milk.

Protein	3.3 g/dL
Fat	3.7 g/dL
Sodium	24 mmol/L

What kind of milk is it?

16.9 A three-year-old boy, who has had recurrent otitis media, is now having difficulties hearing the television. If his right and left ears are equally affected, what would you expect his Rinne and Weber tests to show?

16.10 A 12-year-old, known to have a VSD, has a cardiac catheterization.

RA	81
RV	80
Pulmonary	82
LA	96
LV	90
Aorta	90

What does it show?

16.1   Reactive arthropathy.

Comment: Good response to ibuprofen with no return of symptoms. The ESR can be raised.

16.2   (a) Pubertal response to LHRH stimulation test.

(b) MRI as central cause indicated.

Comment: Remember if LH/FSH is prepubertal, you would have to scan adrenals and ovaries.

16.3   Yes.

Comment: You do not even need to know the test to answer this, as the result is outside the normal range.

16.4   (a) Nephrotic syndrome.

(b) High-dose prednisolone.

(c) Relapsing, but usually remains steroid sensitive.

Comment: You only need to mention fluid management if there is more than one line.

16.5 (a) Renal stone

Nephritic syndrome

Viral cystitis.

(b) Kidney/ureter/bladder X-ray

Urine protein

Blood pressure.

Comment: There is no test for viral cystitis so concentrate on the other two diagnoses.

16.6 (a) Growth hormone deficiency.

(b) Histiocytosis X.

(c) ACTH, TSH studies.

Comment: This is a good example of how (b) and (c) give clues to (a).

16.7 (a) Viral myositis.

(b) He will get better.

Comment: CPK is high enough for muscular dystrophy but unlikely because of the acute onset.

16.8 Cows' milk.

16.9 Both right and left Rinne negative.

Weber central.

16.10 Eisenmenger through the VSD.

Comment: You would lose marks for just Eisenmenger.

Index

63(66) indicates the page reference to a question followed in brackets by the page number to its answer. The reader will often find the condition/disorder is only actually mentioned in the answer. 111(HH) indicates a reference to a 'helpful hint'. The one or two single page references without any brackets refer to material mentioned in an answer without any relevant material in the question.